This fully illustrated atlas and well referenced text provides a comprehensive guide to brain imaging in newborn babies using ultrasound. The volume is unique because it includes examples of normal and abnormal appearances, illustrated from pathological specimens and diagrams of standard views, accompanied by full discussion and advice on prognosis. It also provides an introduction to the physics of ultrasound imaging and Doppler, advice on choosing equipment, guidance on ultrasound safe practice and the care of ill babies during scan examination. Diagnosis of congenital malformations, brain injury and infection is covered, along with a guide to the recognition of artefacts and the appearances of the very immature brain. The volume will be an essential source of reference and guidance for all who work in neonatal intensive care and for radiologists and radiographers.

Neonatal cerebral ultrasound

Neonatal cerebral ultrasound

JANET M. RENNIE MA MD FRCP DCH

Consultant in Neonatal Medicine, Rosie Maternity Hospital, Cambridge
Fellow and Director of Medical Studies, Girton College, Cambridge

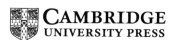

CAMBRIDGE
UNIVERSITY PRESS

PUBLISHED BY THE PRESS SYNDICATE OF THE UNIVERSITY OF CAMBRIDGE
The Pitt Building, Trumpington Street, Cambridge, CB2 1RP, United Kingdom

CAMBRIDGE UNIVERSITY PRESS
The Edinburgh Building, Cambridge, CB2 2RU, United Kingdom
40 West 20th Street, New York, NY 10011-4211, USA
10 Stamford Road, Oakleigh, Melbourne 3166, Australia

First published 1997

Printed in the United Kingdom at the University Press, Cambridge

Typeset in Monotype Ehrhardt 10.5/12 pt

A catalogue record for this book is available from the British Library

Library of Congress Cataloguing in Publication data

Rennie, Janet M.
    Neonatal cerebral ultrasound/Janet M. Rennie.
      p. cm.
    Includes bibliographical references and index.
    ISBN 0 521 45079 9 (hardback)
      1. Ultrasonic encephalography. 2. Infants (Newborn)—Diseases—
Diagnosis. I. Title.
      [DNLM: 1. Cerebrovascular Disorders—in infancy & childhood.
    2. Cerebrovascular Disorders—ultrasonography.
    3. Echoencephalography—in infancy & childhood. 4. Ultrasonography,
    Doppler—in infancy & childhood. WL 355 R416n 1996]
    RJ290.5.R46 1996
    618.92′8047543—dc20   96–13980   CIP
    DNLM/DLC
for Library of Congress

ISBN 0 521 45079 9 hardback

Contents

Preface   viii
Acknowledgements   ix
Glossary   x

1. Principles of ultrasound   1
2. Choice, maintenance and use of equipment   20
3. Normal neonatal cranial ultrasound appearances   38
4. The immature brain   56
5. Monitoring the neonatal brain using Doppler ultrasound   71
6. Vascular lesions I: lesions typical of mature infants   107
7. Vascular lesions II: lesions typical of immature infants   123
8. Enlarged cerebral ventricles   155
9. Infection   170
10. Congenital malformations   177
11. Hypoxic ischaemic encephalopathy   196
12. Cranial ultrasound imaging and prognosis   210
Index   235

Preface

Since the discovery, in 1979, that a real-time image of the neonatal brain could be made through the open anterior fontanelle of the newborn infant, the technique has been widely used to study the brain of vulnerable ill babies. Ultrasound is safe, repeatable, portable and cheap technology, and has therefore become available in most district general hospitals. In many units the technique has become indispensible and is used routinely to image the brain and other organs of infants undergoing intensive care. Junior medial staff and consultants in paediatrics and radiology wish to be able to interpret the results, as the ability to monitor the condition of the brain of babies undergoing intensive care is valuable for prognosis and management. For this reason I have assembled this guide, with an introduction to the basic physics, equipment choice and maintance together with a comprehensive atlas of normal intracranial anatomy with examples of pathological conditions seen in the newborn.

Acknowledgements

As with any book, thanks are due to many: first and foremost to the parents of babies cared for at the Rosie Maternity Hospital, Cambridge, UK and the babies themselves whose (unrecognisable) cranial images form the bulk of the illustrative material. Thanks are also due to a succession of registrars and research fellows who have helped collect material, and to those who have contributed rare examples. Julie Marker, my research assistant from 1991–95, spent hours obtaining obscure references and proof reading. Professor David Evans has been a friend and collaborator for many years and his help with understanding the physics and checking my facts has been invaluable. Malcom Levene's book *Ultrasound of the Infant Brain* (1985) served as an inspiration and as a model; I have drawn on much of his work and am grateful for his support. Lastly, I owe a huge debt of gratitude to my husband, Ian Watts, for his tolerance and encouragement during the long hours I have spent in my study.

Glossary of useful terms

Note: Glossary items appear in italics at first mention in the text

acoustic impedance	the degree of obstruction that a tissue places to the transmission of ultrasound.
acoustic shadow	an area which is poorly visualised with ultrasound due to the fact that most of the beam energy has been reflected by a boundary above it.
aliasing	ambiguity resulting in an erroneous representation of the signal. Results from inadequate sampling, e.g. the fastest velocities appear in the reverse channel when all the flow is forward.
attenuation	loss of energy from the ultrasound beam during its passage through tissue.
axial resolution	the ability to separate two targets along the axis of the beam, that is at different depths in tissue.
boundary	zone partly impermeable to ultrasound, with the ability to reflect and scatter it; may also transmit some.
cavitation	collapse of bubbles under the influence of pressure changes induced by a sound wave.
continuous wave	velocity measuring Doppler system which transmits a beam of ultrasound all the time.
digital (signal)	one represented by a binary 'word' using voltage.
duplex system	the combination of range-gated Doppler velocity estimation superimposed on a real-time image.
energy	measured in Joules per second per square metre, or Watts per square metre. International safety standard maximum of 100 mW.cm^{-2}.
Fourier transform	mathematical technique used in spectral analysis of Doppler signals. Determines component frequencies, a bit like determining the notes in a chord.
Fraunhofer field	the far field away from the transducer; objects subject to distortion in size and can appear fuzzy.
frequency	f; number of cycles per minute; number of times per second that the piezoelectric crystal vibrates.
Fresnel field	the near field of the ultrasound beam; objects clearly focused.
lateral resolution	the ability to distinguish two objects as separate when they are next to each other at the same depth.

linear array	type of ultrasound transducer containing several crystals (often up to 64) in rows.
line density	number of lines per unit distance or degree of arc.
mechanical sector	type of transducer with crystals set on a rotating wheel; easier than rocking them through an arc. Sweep across area of skin contact to give a sector image.
micro streaming	currents set up by variation in size of gas bubbles during the negative phase of the ultrasound cycle.
noise	random fluctuation of signal usually due to electrical interference.
Nyquist limit	the maximum velocity which can be represented without ambiguity using range-gated Doppler; equal to half the pulse repetition frequency.
phased linear array	linear array crystals which are activated electronically in groups producing a sector image.
piezoelectric	description of substance which has the property of generating ultrasound when electrical energy is applied.
pixel	the unit of area of a monitor screen. The number of pixels in part determines the quality of the final image.
pulse-echo	term used in a general way to describe diagnostic imaging machines, as this is how the reflecting boundary is located.
pulse repetition frequency	PRF; the number of bursts of ultrasound each second. Determines the maximum depth in imaging and the maximum velocity measureable in pulsed Doppler mode.
pulsed wave	intermittent beam Doppler system. Allows the depth from which a returning velocity signal came to be determined.
range-gated	the electronic circuitry which allows a Doppler signal to be sampled briefly. Length of the delay allows the depth from which shifted signal came to be determined.
real-time	the description given to a frequently updated image made from passing many beams of ultrasound in slightly different directions, usually presented as a sector, and updating the image about 60 times per sec.
reflection	fate of ultrasound wave which meets a boundary.
refraction	description of fate of the beam which passes through an object in its path and consequently changes in direction.
resolution	the reciprocal distance between two point targets which can just be distinguished with ultrasound.

sample volume	region within the beam from which Doppler signals are analysed.
scattering	what happens to the ultrasound beam when a boundary causes it to break up and travel in many directions.
sonogram	see *spectral analysis*.
spectral analysis	method of presenting the frequencies present within a Doppler shifted spectrum visually.
time-gain compensation	the electronic boosting of information from the far field to compensate for loss of signal by attenuation.
transducer (probe)	converts electrical energy to sound energy, usually via the piezoelectric effect.
velocity	v; of ultrasound in tissue, 1540 m.sec^{-1}. $v = f\lambda$.
wall-thump filter	a filter which eliminates frequencies below 100 Hz from Doppler signals.
wavelength	distance between two identical points of compression on the 'wave' as it passes throught tissue; abbreviated λ.

1   *Principles of ultrasound*

Discovery of Ultrasound

The term ultrasound refers to sound with a frequency above that which can be detected by the human ear. The audible frequency range lies between 20 Hz and 20 kHz (one hertz equals one cycle per second, one kilohertz equals one thousand cycles per second), whereas the frequency of sound waves used for imaging and Doppler applications in medicine are of the order of one thousand times higher than this, with a range between 1 and 10 MHz (M stands for mega, or one million). The existence of sound at a frequency above that which can be heard has been known for hundreds of years; bats use very high pitched sound to detect obstructions. Like audible sound, ultrasound can be reflected from hard surfaces and the returning 'echo' gives the imaging technique its colloquial name. Ultrasound was first exploited by seafarers as 'sonar' (sound navigation and ranging). The pioneers of sonar should also take credit for making the first observations of the biological effects of ultrasound – small fish were killed in the path of the transmitters. During the Second World War, sonar was used to detect submarines and mines beneath ships. By the late 1940s the principles of sonar were being applied to patients. Holmes (1980) graphically described the early imaging investigations – one subject being required to sit in a water filled gun turret with a weight on his abdomen in order for an examination of his neck to be made. Over the next decade, the returning ultrasound echo was used to detect midline shift in head injuries and the presence of foreign bodies in the orbit. Multiple lines of returning echoes could be built up into a two–dimensional picture, and this when frequently updated allows imaging of rapidly moving structures such as heart valves.

Reflection of sound from a moving object gives rise to a change in the observed frequency of the returning sound – the Doppler effect. Christian Doppler was an Austrian physicist who described the phenomenon in 1843. The Doppler effect occurs with light and sound of all wavelengths, and with a knowledge of the transmitted frequency and by measuring the returning frequency one can estimate the velocity of the object involved in making the echo. That this is possible with some accuracy is well known to those who have encountered the Doppler ultrasound speed detectors used by police forces. Gradually, image processing and technology have improved so that now we have a wide range of ultrasound transducers available, often with the addition of colour Doppler to show the direction of blood flow.

Ultrasound waves: basic principles

Ultrasound is emitted from certain special crystals that are able to oscillate at frequencies over a million times per second when energy (mechanical or electrical) is applied to them. These crystals also have the property of detecting received ultrasound and turning it back into electrical energy. Materials include both naturally occuring quartz, cultured lead zirconate and lead titanate. Different crystals have different properties for the propogation and detection of ultrasound. However, the same crystal is used to transmit and receive, sending small bursts of sound energy into the tissue and then 'listening' for the returning waves. Ultrasound for imaging is usually sent out in 'packets' or pulses one or two waves in length.

Ultrasound *energy* spreads by means of compression and rarefaction of molecules, and like sound cannot therefore travel in a vacuum. Gases have too few molecules to ensure reliable transmission of ultrasound waves. The amount of energy contained in the original beam is similar to that of a normal conversation and is gradually dissipated, usually as heat. The energy of ultrasound is measured as the amount in joules transported each second through a square metre. This is usually expressed as $W.m^{-2}$ (one joule per second is one Watt). The ultrasound beam is said to become *attenuated* as energy is lost. The coefficient of attenuation in blood is low, but denser tissues, such as bone, require more energy for the ultrasound to pass through them and may not transmit the energy coherently. This type of tissue thus exhibits high *acoustic impedance* and reflects most of the ultrasound energy directed at it, and also casts an *acoustic shadow* which makes it difficult to image deeper structures. Attenuation is frequency dependent, rising rapidly over the range between 1 and 10 MHz. Intermediate density tissues will reflect and transmit ultrasound, the beam inevitably undergoing a change of direction *(refraction)* as it passes through (Fig. 1.1). The angle of incidence equals the angle of refraction. When the beam encounters an irregular surface it is *scattered* in many directions.

Ultrasound passes through most biological tissue with about the same speed, 1540 metres per second. There is a relationship between the *frequency* of the ultrasound (f) the speed or *velocity* of transmission (v), and the *wavelength* (λ). One wavelength is the distance between two consecutive indentical points on a waveform (Fig. 1.1). The relationship is expressed as:

$$v = \lambda f$$

This equation will become important later in consideration of the smallest object size which it is possible to detect using ultrasound. Further reading on the physics of ultrasound can be found in the book edited by McDicken (1991).

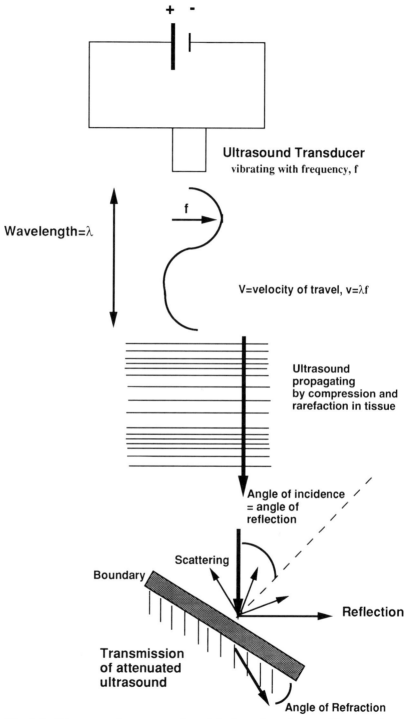

Fig. 1.1. *Diagrammatic representation of the fate of an ultrasound beam in tissue.*

Echo location

The key to placing the depth of the returned echo is measuring the time which the energy takes to return to the crystal. Because the speed of ultrasound in tissue is known to be fairly constant, the simple equation:

$$\text{distance} = \text{velocity} \times \text{time}$$

can be used to calculate the depth from which the reflected energy came. Measuring the elapsed time will give rise to an estimate exactly double the depth of the object within the tissue as the ultrasound has to travel out and back before time is measured (Fig. 1.2). After a pulse of ultrasound energy has been transmitted it is likely that several returned pulses will be sensed at different times, as reflections occur from the various structures which the beam encounters. Eventually the energy will be completely dissipated and no more will return. Loss of energy and the time which is allowed to elapse between sucessive pulses will limit the maximum depth which it is possible to interrogate. As a guide, it is possible to penetrate roughly 200 wavelengths through the tissue. The imaging technique thus depends on *pulse-echo*, and this term is often used to describe imaging with ultrasound.

Methods of displaying located echo information

A-mode

The simplest method of displaying the results obtained by passing a beam of ultrasound into tissue and receiving the 'echo' from the same plane of tissue is with the use of a cathode ray oscilloscope screen to display the amplitude of the returning signal. The earliest peak represents ultrasound reflected from near the surface and the amount of sound reflected will vary according to the acoustic properties of the tissue. This is the old 'A-mode' or amplitude mode used to detect midline shift (see Fig. 1.2). A-mode is very rarely used now although some modern commercial equipment offers the information as an addition to the *real-time* display.

B-mode and real-time imaging: types of transducer

Instead of plotting the returned sound as a peak, the contained amplitude information is converted into a degree of brightness (hence B mode) and placed on the screen at a distance representing the depth from which the returned sound came. Calculation of the depth is done by measuring elapsed time, as already explained above. By building up information obtained from many pulses of ultrasound sent in different directions through the tissue, holding the degree of brightness in short-term memory and allowing the information to persist for a short time on the screen, a grey scale picture can be built up. This can be achieved either from up to 200 *piezoelectric* crystals mounted in rows on a single head *(linear array)*

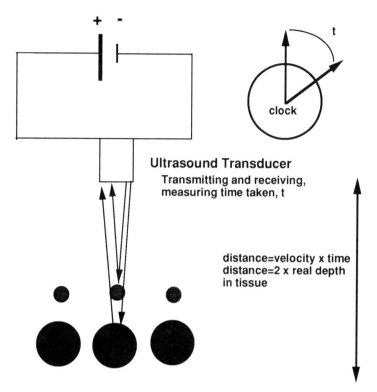

Ultrasound Transducer
Transmitting and receiving,
measuring time taken, t

distance=velocity x time
distance=2 x real depth
in tissue

Display of information received by transducer

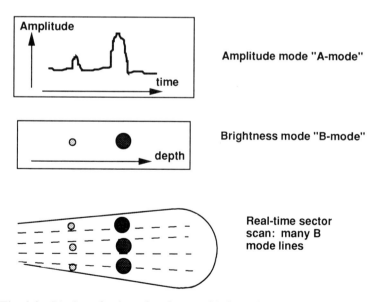

Amplitude mode "A-mode"

Brightness mode "B-mode"

Real-time sector
scan: many B
mode lines

Fig. 1.2. *Display of pulse–echo ultrasound information.*

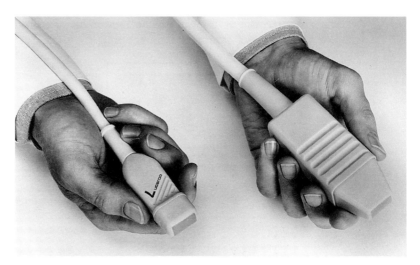

Fig. 1.3. *Ultrasound transducers with small footprints suitable for examination of the neonatal brain. (Courtesy of Acuson.)*

or from two or three elements that can rotate on a wheel inside the *transducer* head *(mechanical sector)*. The movement of the transducers can be done electronically or mechanically, and linear array transducers with large numbers of crystals are often computer activated in different groups – *phased linear array*. The image produced by phased linear array or mechanical sector transducers is an arc of a circle. The size of the arc, or sector, is determined by the most peripheral point on the skin with which the transducer can make contact, and by the amount of information which is needed to build up and retain the image. One line per degree of arc maintains a reasonable image. This type of equipment is often termed a 2-D sector scanner. Updating the image many times per second allows changes in position of even rapidly moving objects such as heart valves to be shown as in real time. Changes in the position of organs due to respiration or vascular pulsation are easily seen. More than 25 images per second are required to prevent 'flicker' and usual frame rates are 60 per second. Each sector image contains between 50 and 150 separate B-mode lines and is updated line-by-line so that the beam appears to 'sweep' across the tissue. The speed of ultrasound in tissue is so fast that each line of information is acquired in less than 1 msec. A small 'footprint' or area which is in contact with the skin is useful for neonatal examinations in view of the curvature of the head. Figure 1.3 illustrates a small linear array transducer suitable for imaging the neonatal brain.

Limits of resolution of ultrasound

Many factors influence the smallest size of object that can be successfully resolved with ultrasound. The operator plays a vital role in choosing the best transducer for the job, in setting the sensitivity and gain controls correctly and using coupling gel properly to eliminate loss of ultrasound before the skin surface. The sector arc can be made smaller to increase the *line density*. Performance can be checked with various commercially produced phantoms and test objects and these are discussed in Chapter 2. Machine-based factors include the amount of electrical *noise* present in the system, the power, the beam width and the wavelength. As the velocity of ultrasound in biological tissue is relatively constant, to obtain ultrasound of smaller wavelength requires higher frequency transducers. The wavelength of ultrasound transmitted through the body from a 1 MHz transducer is 1.5 mm, and hence from a 10 MHz transducer 0.15 mm. Transducers with a high frequency are capable of resolving smaller parts; for the neonatal brain a 7.5 MHz transducer is now usually chosen, and most of the pictures in this book were taken using a probe of this frequency. The reason why 10 MHz transducers are not used all the time is that the depth of penetration into tissue is less with very high frequency transducers, because the energy contained is dissipated (attenuated) more easily. In biological soft tissue the attenuation coefficient is roughly proportional to the frequency. The depth of penetration of a 10 MHz transducer with energy 100 mW.cm^{-2} is about 20 cm, whereas a 5 MHz probe transmitting similar energy will reach tissue at 40 cm. In practice, therefore, the choice of probe is a compromise between the depth of the image required and the desire for a high degree of *resolution* with the least power output according to the type of tissue being imaged.

Axial resolution

Resolution has been defined as the reciprocal of the distance between two point targets which can just be distinguished apart. *Axial resolution* refers to the ability to distinguish objects which are close to each other or lying one behind the other in the axis of the beam, that is parallel to the direction of the ultrasound. Axial resolving capacity is much better than that achieved for *lateral resolution*, and this is a good reason for carrying out ultrasound examinations in two planes wherever possible. The factors which determine axial resolution include the duration of the echo pulse, the wavelength and the settings of the ultrasound machine. In a perfect machine, axial resolution is equal to half the pulse length. Raju & Zikos (1987) quote an axial resolution of 0.7 mm and a lateral resolution of 1.6 mm using a 5 MHz probe to image the neonatal brain.

Lateral resolution

The wavelength of ultrasound is not the only factor influencing the ability to measure and distinguish small objects. The beam of ultrasound that travels into the tissue starts out the same size as the crystal, which is usually disc-shaped. The beam thus resembles torchlight, and like a beam of light it diverges as it travels. The cylindrical portion of the beam near to the transducer where resolution is good is termed the *Fresnel field*, and the far field where distortion and fuzziness are likely is termed the *Fraunhofer field*. The ultrasound beam can be focused with acoustic lenses (or by manufacturing the crystal with a concave surface) in order to improve the precision of measurement for objects that are at the same depth, at right angles to the path of the beam. This ability is termed lateral resolution, and is always less good than axial resolution. The best lateral resolution is achieved with a narrow well-focused beam with a long near field, hence the need for high frequencies and the compromise between the desire for high resolution and low power referred to above.

Contrast resolution

This is the ability of an image to display different shades of grey representing different tissue reflectivity. The final image is affected by reflected and scattered echoes from many different targets and the contrast resolution is thus degraded. The speckled pattern of a typical real-time ultrasound image results from signal fluctuation or noise and reduces the ability to depict small contrast changes. The capability of the equipment as a whole must be considered; the returning electrical information undergoes much processing before the image is presented, usually on a television monitor. At this point the number of *pixels*, or dots, which make up the screen is the final arbiter of the ability to make out and measure small objects separately from each other. The quality of signal processing affects speckle reduction and interference from noise. In practice, a good quality 7.5 MHz imaging transducer operating on the infant head is capable of resolving about 1 or 2 mm lateral resolution, a performance a good deal worse than that which would be predicted from the wavelength alone. For comparison, magnetic resonance imaging or a good quality computed tomography (CT) image with 512 pixels would resolve about 0.5 mm. These techniques do not suffer from the attenuation problems of ultrasound.

Temporal resolution

This is defined as the minimum separation in time for which two events can be observed (McDicken, 1991). The time interval between one frame and the next is about 40 msec with a frame rate of 25 per second. Events occuring faster than this, such as flutter of heart valves, could therefore be missed. The time taken to build up a complete sector image is about 40 msec so that events which appear on the same image have not all taken place simultaneously.

Improving the image: time-gain compensation and suppression

Apart from attempting to improve resolution with beam focusing, the ability of ultrasound to image deep structures can be improved by enhancing the echoes returning from the far field and supressing those returning

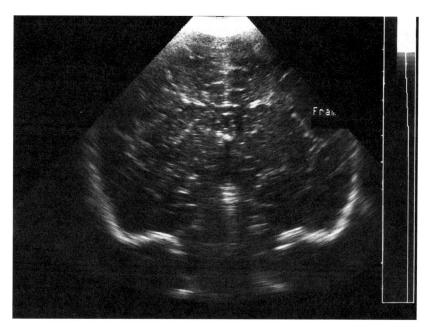

Fig. 1.4. *Ultrasound scan picture with time-gain compensation applied to the signal; note graphical display of slope at the right-hand side of the picture.*

from the near field. Electronic circuitry is used to boost or give 'gain' to the longer-returning echoes, hence the term *time-gain compensation* or TGC. Manufacturers divide the field into sections and give the operator the opportunity to adjust the compensation for each depth individually in order to give the best image possible. The 'slope' or amount of boost for each setting can often be displayed at the side of the image for information. Figure 1.4 shows the information displayed as a line graph alongside a black-and-white image to which varying TGC has been applied. Automatic TCG is possible, and if this is available the ultrasound machine sets the gain according to the strength of the returning echoes.

Suppression (rejection) of weak returning echoes helps to enhance the image, as often these are due to artefact. When setting up the sensitivity controls at the start of imaging, suppression and TCG are best adjusted to low levels. The overall gain or power can then be set to give a suitable reflection from the main object of interest, the other controls are then refined to supress unwanted small echoes and enhance areas of interest. Many machines offer the ability to preserve in the computer's memory the combinations of settings which produce the best result for an individual structure.

Estimating the velocity of a moving target with ultrasound: the Doppler effect

So far we have considered the behaviour of ultrasound waves with regard to static *boundaries* within tissues. However, any energy wave may encounter a moving target which is also capable of reflecting the beam, and ultrasound is no exception. Christian Doppler described the effect of transmitting sound from a moving target, when as the object moves towards the observer the wavelength is 'squashed' thus raising the pitch of the sound, and as the sound source moves away the wavelength is lengthened lowering the pitch. The phenomenon is an everyday one, common examples being the noise of trains rushing through stations and the effect on the tone of ambulance sirens as they pass by. Astronomers have exploited the change in wavelength of light caused by movement of stars. In medicine, the Doppler effect has been of most value in the estimation of the velocity of blood flowing in vessels. More recently a semi-quantitative application has been developed in order to colour-code the movement of blood and superimpose the colour onto the real-time grey scale image. As an aside, because the term Doppler effect refers to a proper name it should always be written with an initial capital letter.

The Doppler equation

More information on the pitfalls involved in velocity calculations is contained in Chapter 6, and much more detail on the whole topic in the book by Evans *et al.* (1989). When an ultrasound beam of transmitted frequency (f_t) encounters a moving target the reflected frequency (f_r) is changed by an amount f_d. The relationship can be expressed in the following equation:

$$f_d = (f_t - f_r) = f_t \; \frac{2v \cos \theta}{c}$$

where v is the velocity of the target, θ the angle between the ultrasound beam and the direction of motion of the target and c the velocity of sound in the tissue. To estimate the velocity requires only that both f_t and f_r and the angle of insonation are measured as c is known. A small angle of insonation mean that cos θ is close to 1. Hence to obtain the most accurate result when measuring velocity with Doppler ultrasound it is important to insonate the target with the beam pointing directly at it, like looking down the barrel of a gun. The cosine of an angle varies a great deal at values around 90°. This means that a small error of estimation for angles of insonation above 60° gives rise to a relatively large error in the velocity calculation. Although angle corrections are therefore possible, they should be avoided.

Types of Doppler ultrasound transducer

Ultrasound is generated either all the time by the transducer in a *continuous wave* (CW), or in bursts a few wavelengths long in a *pulsed wave* (PW) system. Continuous wave Doppler systems have a transmitting and a receiving crystal, and a combination of filters and amplifiers is used to extract the Doppler shifted signal from the returning ultrasound. This process is known as demodulation. By chance, the velocity of blood flow means that the shifted frequency falls within the audible range and can be presented as an audio signal. Directional analysis of flow towards and away from the probe can be presented in different channels of stereo headphones and recorded onto audio tape for further processing. The human ear is a sensitive instrument and the fact that Doppler signals can be heard in this way has undoubtedly helped the success of the method, as a trained operator can gain a great deal of information just by listening. Blood flow in a vessel occurs with more than one velocity and the changes induced by diseased or stenosed segments often produce a characteristic pattern of noise that can be detected by ear. However, more objective analysis and the conversion of the information into a form that can be represented pictorially requires *spectral analysis*.

Duplex systems

The disadvantages of continuous wave systems include the lack of spatial precision as it is impossible to know the depth at which the change in frequency occurred, and the fact that the returning ultrasound may have undergone a change induced by more than one moving target. These disadvantages are overcome by pulsed wave Doppler in which a single crystal transmits ultrasound in short bursts. By limiting the time for which the crystal is 'listening' for returning sound, only that coming from a certain depth will be sampled. The signal is thus *'range-gated'*. The combination of pulsed wave Doppler and a real-time B-scan system is a powerful investigative tool as velocities can be sampled from known anatomical locations (Fig. 1.5). This type of equipment is termed a *duplex system*. The ability to range-gate the signal enables a small *sample volume* to be used to estimate the velocity accurately.

Maximum velocity limit of duplex systems

Range-gated duplex systems have one major drawback; they are only able to detect velocities unambiguously up to a finite maximum. Very fast-moving particles may pass right through the area of sampling between transmission of sucessive pulses if the gap is too long, being 'missed' altogether by the sampling beam. Shannon (1949) stated that it was necessary to sample a signal to at least twice the highest frequency present to avoid ambiguity. The maximum Doppler shift that can be detected is half the *pulse repetition frequency* (PRF), and this is known as the Nyquist frequency. The corresponding maximum velocity, which can be obtained by inserting this value into the Doppler equation, is termed the *Nyquist limit*. The Nyquist limit will vary with the depth setting; when deep structures are examined enough time must be allowed for the pulses to make the round journey and hence only slow velocities can be sampled. If the Nyquist limit is exceeded the phenomenon of *aliasing* will occur, when the highest velocities are represented in the reverse channel (Fig. 1.6).

11

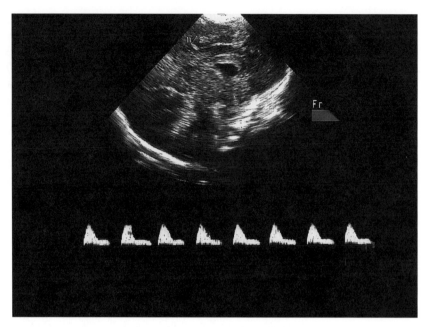

Fig. 1.5. *Duplex Doppler output; system allows measurement of velocity information in a specified position within the image depth. Note display of the information as a sonogram after signal processing.*

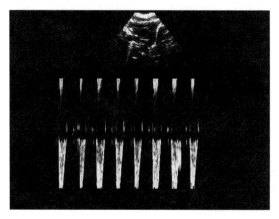

Fig. 1.6. *Example of aliasing range-gated Doppler velocity information. Tops of velocity profiles appear in the reverse channel.*

Aliasing

An analogy can be made between aliasing in a Doppler ultrasound signal and that which occurs when filming a rotating wheel; if sampling (the frame rate of the film) is not done often enough the wheel may turn through almost two revolutions, then not quite four and so on so that in the resulting series of sampled images it appears to travel backwards – a far from true representation of what actually happened. Aliasing is such an important problem of range–gated Doppler that all users owe it to their patients to be on the lookout for it. The example represented in Fig. 1.6 would be fairly easy to spot, but if the aliasing is very marked the Doppler signal can 'wrap around' the forward and reverse channels making the resulting display appear like that of turbulent flow. If there is a possibility that aliasing is occuring it is possible to check, either by using continuous wave ultrasound with which aliasing cannot occur, or by increasing the PRF. Increasing the PRF introduces some range ambiguity, however, as it is always possible that whilst the gate is open the sampled frequencies contain some from the last pulse which has travelled twice as far as the intended depth of interrogation. With a high PRF two or more significant 'gates' may exist and for this reason this solution is not used routinely to overcome the problem of aliasing. In the extreme case with a very high PRF, pulsed wave Doppler becomes like a continuous wave in that high velocities can be measured accurately but there is no range resolution.

Doppler signal processing

The Doppler shifted signals returned from sampling a typical blood vessel with many ultrasound pulses contain many different frequencies, as not all blood corpuscles within it are moving at the same velocity. The complexity of the returned signal requires signal processing, both for audio interpretation and visual presentation as a sonogram. Apart from amplification it is customary to subject the signal to a filter to remove interference. This filter is often called a *wall-thump filter*, because high-amplitude low-velocity signals arise from the movement of the blood vessel rather than the blood within it. Wall-thump filters are usually set between 100 and 500 Hz, giving rise to a gap in the spectrum of velocities around zero. This can give rise to inaccuracies when distinguishing between minor degrees of reversed diastolic flow, and for neonatal cerebral work it is important to set the filter as low as possible. Further electronic circuitry is involved in unscrambling forward and reverse flow, and in order to provide a sonogram. Early attempts at providing a written objective record of the audio signal, which could be transferred between units, involved the zero crossing detector. This type of signal processsor functions by counting the number of times a signal crosses its own mean value in a given time; unfortunately its performance is particularly poor when a large number of frequencies are involved and these frequency processors are highly subject to interference from noise. They are still incorporated into some equipment because of their low cost, but should be avoided. The best method of signal processing is spectral analysis. This involves performing a *Fourier transform* to determine all the frequencies present in a few milliseconds of returning ultrasound (like resolving which notes are present in a musical chord) and presenting the information with a grey scale representing the power of the signal (the loudness of each note). Successive 'quanta' of milliseconds of information are analysed and presented one after another, building up in time along the X axis, with frequency along the Y axis. The resulting sonogram is a familiar feature of duplex systems, but the computer power required adds considerably to the cost. Further reduction of information is required for velocity estimation and is discussed in Chapter 6.

Colour Doppler

The combination of multiple Doppler samples across a real-time image can be used to provide a velocity profile over a wide area, and the concept of colour-coding the velocity information was first proposed in 1981 (Eyer *et al.*, 1981). Now real-time colour flow mapping (CFM) systems are commonplace. The usual pulse-echo B scan is used to provide a grey scale image and multiple Doppler interrogations are performed in order to provide information about the direction and velocity of blood flow in the same area. Colour flow mapping is perhaps of most use in cardiology, but the application of colour to a real-time image can show the situation of vessels, speeding up the time taken to obtain Doppler signals from neonatal cranial arteries (Plate 1.1). Abnormal vascular leashes can be seen, allowing the diagnosis of arterio-venous malformations. Colour Doppler is only roughly quantitative; the colour scale is applied by comparing the velocity at any given point to a 'memory bank' of velocities and then colouring the image with shades of red through to yellow for flow towards the transducer and shades of blue through to purple for flow away from it. Manufacturers often cite that 128 shades of colour are applied, although in practice the operator can only distinguish four or five. Turbulent flow is represented as green, and colour aliasing can occur with very high velocities in the same way as described for range-gated Doppler. Aliasing can result in fast flow being coded as green (turbulent) when in fact it has just not been sampled often enough. Turbulent jets should therefore be checked, as advised for possible aliasing, with continuous wave Doppler ultrasound.

Safety: physical and biological effects of ultrasound

Sound waves are a form of energy, and the energy levels involved in ultrasound imaging are similar to those of normal conversation, and 100 times less than those used for ultrasound diathermy. However, the addition of colour Doppler has meant that the time taken to perform a diagnostic scan has lengthened recently and the possibility of biological effects occuring at the energy levels used has been re-explored. Energy output is measured in $mW.cm^{-2}$, and the American Institute for Ultrasound in Medicine (AIUM, 1988) has set a maximum acceptable level for the peak output of $100\ mW.cm^{-2}$. The output of several commercial pulsed Doppler units can reach levels of $500–1000\ mW.cm^{-2}$. It is important that operators are aware of the output from the machine they use regularly (see Chapter 2) and

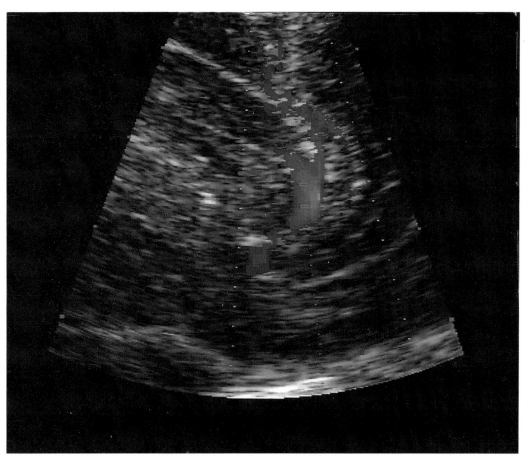

Plate 1.1 *Example of colour flow mapping in the neonatal brain. The anterior cerebral artery appears red; flow towards the transducer.*

keep the time of examination to the minimum, particularly when using colour or pulsed Doppler. There are three main types of physical effect: heating, streaming and cavitation, and these together with vibration effects on large molecules constitute the major areas of concern (Baker & Dalrymple, 1978; Nyborg & Ziskin, 1985). Distortion of the waveform could occur due to minor variations in the speed of transmission in tisssue of different density, and theoretically this could give rise to a shock wave (Duck & Starritt, 1984). Shock waves arise more readily in water, and the possibility needs to be taken into consideration when ultrasound is transmitted through a fluid path. Shock waves are produced deliberately in the ultrasound lithotripters which are used to destroy renal stones, and these can certainly cause *cavitation*.

Heating

Ultrasound is attenuated as it passes through tissue, most of the energy being dissipated as heat. Heating has not been observed to occur in mammalian tissue at diagnostic levels, and is not thought to present a practical problem as the body has efficient mechanisms for accommodating changes in temperature. Using 3 MHz ultrasound at energy levels of 3000 mW.cm^{-2}, haemolysis could be induced *in vivo* (Williams *et al.*, 1986), and this high energy level could result in a temperature rise of several degrees Celsius if applied to tissues for 5 minutes. Diagnostic imaging of the fetus has been calculated to produce a temperature rise less than one degree Celsius. Some concern has been raised about local 'hot spots' damaging individual cells, but there is no evidence that these occur.

Cavitation and streaming

Most ordinary liquids contain stable microbubbles, as does some plant and insect tissue. These can grow during the negative pressure phase of the ultrasound cycle, and if they are made to resonate they can cause local currents to be set up – this is termed *micro-streaming*. Under certain conditions it may be possible for undissolved gas bubbles to give rise to the same effect. Micro-streaming has been shown to disrupt cells, including erythrocytes (Gershoy & Nyborg, 1973; Miller & Williams, 1983; Canstensen *et al.*, 1993) and may disrupt macromolecules and change membrane permeability or charge (Dino *et al.*, 1989). Sound waves can result in standing waves if they are reflected back and forth between parallel surfaces, and marked resonance can occur if the separation of the surfaces is half a wavelength. Dyson *et al.* (1974) set up standing waves in the circulation of the chick embryo using ultrasound of 1–5 MHz, 12 W.cm^{-2} for 15 minutes. It has been suggested that bubbles in blood could be driven to resonate (Fairbank & Scully, 1977). Cavitation describes the creation and rapid growth of a bubble which bursts, and this phenomenon has been described *in vivo* with therapeutic but not diagnostic levels of ultrasound (ter Haar & Daniels, 1981). The high local energy densities within collapsing voids may result in free radical release (Carmichael *et al.*, 1986). Microbubbles have fortunately not been shown to exist in blood, and Williams was unable to produce cavitation even in artificially injected bubbles (Williams *et al.*, 1985). However, it is not possible to state categorically at this stage that cavitation never occurs in biological tissue, and this group of biological effects are the most important.

Chromosome disruption

The possibility of chromosome damage due to vibration of DNA has been raised, and the work of Liebeskind *et al.* (1979a,b, 1981) received much attention. Others have not been able to replicate these effects (Boyd *et al.*, 1971), nor have there been consistent reports of increased sister chromatid exchanges, a more sensitive test for chromosome damage (Goss, 1984). Harrison & Baker-Kubiczek (1991) were unable to demonstrate neoplastic transformation in mouse embryo fibroblasts, and the overall expert view is that these effects have been overstated (Wells, 1987).

Epidemiological surveys

Perhaps the most convincing evidence for the safety of ultrasound with relevance to neonatal practice comes from the large surveys of the results of diagnostic imaging in pregnancy. Several large-scale surveys have recently been reported, and there has been a suggestion that more infants are left-handed after exposure to ultrasound *in utero* (Salvesen *et al.*, 1993) and one study which reported an increased incidence of growth retardation (Newnham *et al.*, 1993). Although growth retardation, reduced fetal movements and a lower white cell count have been shown in primate fetuses exposed many times to ultrasound *in utero* (Tarantal & Hendrickx, 1989) these effects have not been consistent in humans (Wladimiroff & Laar, 1980; Bakketeig *et al.*, 1984; Stark *et al.*, 1984) and in general there is considered to be no evidence for adverse effects of ultrasound exposure (Ziskin & Petitti, 1988).

Reports and recommendations of professional organisations

The World Health Organisation, the AIUM, the European Federation of Societies for Ultrasound in Medicine and Biology and the Japanese Society of Ultrasonics have all evaluated the literature regarding safety (Kossof & Nyborg, 1989). The overwhelming conclusion is that there are no confirmed deleterious effects of diagnostic ultrasound. The guidelines for the upper limit of safe output remain 100 mW.cm^{-2}, although this level cannot be a guarantee as the reports acknowledge the lack of reliable human data regarding relatively prolonged, low intensity exposure. Most manufacturers allow their equipment to exceed the guideline output, and leave the decision regarding the use of higher power to the user. The prudent operator will attempt to limit the exposure of his or her patient to a minimum, and a significant reduction can be achieved by following these simple suggestions (modified from Evans *et al.*, 1989, with permission):

1. Use the lowest transmitted power that will give a result.
2. Keep the duration of the examination to a minimum.
3. Use CW Doppler rather than PW if it will give a result.
4. Use the lowest PRF of pulsed Doppler that will allow the highest velocity to be measured.
5. Do not leave the Doppler beam irradiating a particular region for longer than is necessary. Switch back to imaging mode as soon as the Doppler examination is complete.
6. Use colour Doppler only when necessary to make the diagnosis.

References

AIUM (American Institute of Ultrasound in Medicine) (1988) Bioeffects considerations for the safety of diagnostic ultrasound. *Journal of Ultrasound in Medicine*, 7 (Suppl.).

Baker, M.L. & Dalrymple, G.V. (1978) Biological effects of diagnostic ultrasound: a review. *Radiology*, 126:479–83.

Bakketeig, L.S., Eik-Nes, S.H. & Jacobsen, G. *et al.* (1984) Randomised controlled tiral of ultrasonographic screening in pregnancy. *Lancet*, ii:207–11.

Boyd, E., Abdulla, U., Donald, I., Fleming, J.E.E., Hall, A.J. & Ferguson-Smith, M.A. (1971) Chromosome breakage and ultrasound. *British Medical Journal*, 2:501–2.

Canstensen, E. L. (1993) Lysis of erythrocytes by exposure to ultrasound. *Ultrasound in Medicine and Biology* 19:147

Carmichael, A.J., Mosoba, M.M., Riesz, P. & Christman, C.L. (1986) Free radical production in aqueous solutions exposed to simulated ultrasonic diagnostic conditions. *IEEE Transactions on Ultrasonics, Ferroelectrics and Frequency Control, UFFC*, 33:148–55.

Dino, M.A., Dyson, M., Young, S.R., Mortimer, A.J., Hart, J. & Crum, L.A. (1989) The significance of membrane change in the safe and effective use of therapeutic and diagnostic ultrasound. *Physics in Medicine and Biology*, 34: 1543–52.

Duck, F.A. & Starritt, H.C. (1984) Acoustic shock generation by ultrasonic imaging equipment. *British Journal of Radiology*, 57:231–40.

Dyson, M., Pond, J.B., Woodward, B. & Broadbent, J. (1974) The production of blood cell stasis and endothelial damage in blood vessels of chick embryos treated with ultrasound in a stationary wave. *Ultrasound in Medicine and Biology*, 1:133–48.

Evans, D.H., McDicken, W.N., Skidmore, R. & Woodcock, J.P. (1989) *Doppler Ultrasound: Physics, Instrumentation and Clinical Applications*. Chichester: John Wiley & Sons Ltd.

Eyer, M.K., Brandestini, M.A., Phillips, D.J. & Baker, D.W. (1981) Colour digital echo/Doppler image presentation. *Ultrasound in Medical Biology*, 7:21–31.

Fairbank, W.M. & Scully, M.O. (1977) A new noninvasive technique for cardiac pressure measurement: resonant scattering of ultrasound from bubbles. *IEEE Transactions on Biomedical Engineering BME*, 24:107–10.

Gershoy, A. & Nyborg, W.L. (1973) Pertubation of plant-cell contents by ultrasonic micro-irradiation. *Journal of the Acoustic Society of America*, **54**:1356–67.

Goss, S.A. (1984) Sister chromatid exchange and ultrasound. *Journal of Ultrasound in Medicine*, **3**:463–70.

Harrison, G.H. & Baker-Kubiczek, E.K. (1991) Pulsed ultrasound and neoplastic transformation *in vitro*. *Ultrasound in Medicine and Biology*, **17**:627–32.

Holmes, J.H. (1980) Ultrasound during the early years of AIUM. *Journal of Clinical Ultrasound*, **8**:299–308.

Kossof, G. & Nyborg, W.L. (Eds.) (1989) World federation of ultrasound in medicine and biology. Symposium on safety and standardisation in medical ultrasound. *Ultrasound in Medicine and Biology*, **15** (suppl 1).

Liebeskind, D., Bases, R., Elequin, F., Neubort, S., Leifer, R., Goldberg, R. & Koenigsberg, M. (1979a) Diagnostic ultrasound: effects on the DNA and gowth patterns of animal cells. *Radiology*, **131**:77–184.

Liebeskind, D., Bases, R., Mendez, F., Elequin, F. & Koenigsberg, M. (1979b) Sister chromatid exchanges in human lymphocytes after exposure to Doppler ultrasound. *Science*, **205**:1273–5.

Liebeskind, D., Koenigsberg, M., Koss, L. & Raventos, C. (1981) Morphological changes in the surface characteristics of cultured cells after exposure to diagnostic ultrasound. *Radiology*, **138**:419–23.

McDicken, W.N. (1991) *Diagnostic Ultrasonics*, 3rd edn. Edinburgh: Churchill Livingstone.

Miller, D.L. & Williams, A.R. (1983) Further investigations of ATP release from human erythrocytes exposed to ultrasonically activated gas-filled pores. *Ultrasound in Medicine and Biology*, **9**:297–307.

Newnham, J.P., Evans, S.F., Michael, C.A., Stanley, F.J. & Landau, L.I. (1993) Effects of frequent ultrasound during pregnancy: a randomised controlled trial. *Lancet*, **342**: 887–91.

Nyborg, W.L. & Ziskin, M.C. (Eds.) (1985) *Biological Effects of Ultrasound*. New York: Churchill Livingstone.

Raju, T.N.K. & Zikos, E. (1987) Regional cerebral blood flow velocity in infants – a real time transcranial and fontanellar pulsed Doppler study. *Journal of Ultrasound in Medicine*, **6**:497–507.

Salvesen, K.A., Vatten, L.J., Eik-Nes, S.H., Hugdahl, K. & Bakketeig, L.S. (1993) Routine ultrasonography in utero and subsequent handedness and neurological development. *British Medical Journal*, **307**:159–64.

Shannon, C.E. (1949) Communications in the presence of noise. *Proc IRE* **37**:10–21.

Stark, C.R., Orleans, M., Haverkamp, A.D. & Murphy, J. (1984) Short and long term risks after exposure to diagnostic ultrasound in utero. *Obstetrics and Gynaecology*, **63**:194–200.

Tarantal, A.F. & Hendrickx, A.G. (1989) Evaluation of the bioeffects of prenatal ultrasound exposure in the Cynomolgus Macaque (*Macaca fascicularis*): I. Neonatal/infant observations. *Teratology* **39**:137–47.

ter Haar, G. & Daniels, S. (1981) Evidence for ultrasonically induced cavitation *in vivo*. *Physics in Medicine and Biology*, **26**:1145–9.

Wells, P.N.T. (1987) The safety of diagnostic ultrasound. *British Journal of Radiology*, **20** (Suppl.)

Williams, A.R., Gross, D.R. & Miller, D.L. (1985) Cavitation in mammalian blood: an *in vivo* search. In: *Proceedings of the 4th Meeting of the World Federation of Ultrasound in Medicine and Biology*, ed. R.W. Gill & M.J. Dadd, p. 484. Sydney: Pergamon Press.

Williams, A.R., Miller, D.L. & Gross, D.R. (1986) Haemolysis *in vivo* by therapeutic intensities of ultrasound. *Ultrasound in Medical Biology*, **12**:501–9.

Wladimiroff, J.W. & Laar, J. (1980) Ultrasonic measurement of fetal body size. *Acta Obstetrica Gynaecologica Scandinavica*, **59**:177–9.

Ziskin, M.C. & Petitti, D.B. (1988) Epidemiology of human exposure to ultrasound: a critical review. *Ultrasound in Medicine and Biology*, **14**:91–96.

2 *Choice, maintenance and use of equipment*

Introduction

There is a vast range of suitable equipment available for neonatal ultrasound, and the relatively low price has made it possible for many neonatal units to have their own, dedicated machine. This has many advantages for the sick neonate who can then undergo diagnostic imaging without waiting or being moved from the incubator. A readily available machine allows ultrasound to be used for research and audit without the concerns which would be raised regarding the ethics of transporting a severely ill baby to acquire such information. A single unit can be chosen which will allow cardiac, hip and abdominal work to be carried out in addition to cranial ultrasound scanning, and for this reason many busy neonatal intensive care units can justify the additional cost of colour Doppler which facilitates cardiac diagnosis. If cardiac imaging is not to be undertaken then the additional cost of both colour and CW/PW Doppler may not be worthwhile as in most other regions of the body a good quality black and white image will suffice. When evaluating new equipment it helps to remember that a neonatal machine will be used mainly for monochrome imaging, and that revolving three-dimensional reconstructions in colour will not compensate for poor image quality. A good basic system can be put together for less than £20,000 (at 1995 prices). Most systems can be upgraded should colour or CW/PW Doppler become necessary. This chapter cannot be comprehensive but aims to provide a few pointers for those who are contemplating purchase. There is no substitute for personally trying out new equipment. Most manufacturers are only too willing to arrange a trial, and often provide some training.

On-line database of ultrasound equipment

The University of Glasgow, UK, maintains a database of diagnostic medical ultrasound equipment which is available to anyone with access to a personal computer and a modem via the internet or the joint academic network (JANET). Information from the manufacturers is stored in a standardised format and systems grouped into different categories. Users of the database should be able to quickly and easily identify potentially suitable equipment and suppliers. A connection must first be made to the University of Glasgow information system, GLANCE. The way to make the connection depends on the communications equipment and software, but the connection address is *info.glasgow.uk.ac*. It may be possible to call this from your local network, alternatively the direct dial–up number is 0141 334 8100 using a modem speed of 2400 baud. Using Telenet or Gopher software call *telenet info.gla.ac.uk* or *gopher info.gla.ac.uk* which will take you directly into GLANCE. Once connected to GLANCE type *info* to connect, and the Ultrasound Equipment Evaluation Project (UEEP) can be accessed using a menu route via the following tree. From the first menu choose:

11. Subject-based information service,
then choose,
15. Medicine and Health,
then
1. Ultrasound Equipment Evaluation Project
and finally
2. UEEP Medical Ultrasound Equipment database.

Further information can be obtained by contacting the University of Glasgow, see Table 2.1 for details.

Guidelines regarding available equipment

This area moves so fast that a prospective purchaser would be well advised to consult the UEEP database mentioned above. The range of equipment begins with the small, almost 'table top' scanners such as the Aloka SSD-500, the Toshiba Capasee (SSA-220A), Siel Imaging's SDU-350, Dynamic Imaging's Concept series or the Pie Medical 200 (Fig. 2.1). For a price of around £13,000 (at 1995 prices) these scanners do not offer colour or PW/CW Doppler but produce a reliable, good quality monochrome image. Their size and price makes them an attractive option for crowded neonatal units. The availability of a small, light 7.5 MHz probe suitable for imaging neonatal heads (Fig. 1.3) is not universal and is something to ask about when considering purchase. Higher up the range, a black and white system with a printer such as the Hewlett Packard HP Sonos 100CF or Advanced Technology Laboratories (ATL) Ultramark 4 would cost around £20,000 (at 1995 prices); the former is upgradable to include colour flow and CW/PW Doppler.

Top of the range systems cost much more but ultrasound technology is still cheap when compared to other imaging equipment. 'Gold standard' equipment such as the Acuson 128XP (Fig. 2.2), the Toshiba SSH-140HG or the ATL Apogee 800 cost around £80,000–100,000 (at 1995 prices) but all offer excellent rapidly refreshed imaging with zoom and review, colour Doppler, PW/CW Doppler, and full storage and retrieval facilities. With the increasing importance of neuroimaging results in litigation, this is becoming vital. When studying information remember that the probe and peripherals are usually costed separately. There are often other ultrasound

Table 2.1. *Contact information for the major ultrasound manufacturers (UK, European and US addresses are included where available)*

Company	Address	Telephone & Fax
Acuson	Lakeside House, Stockley Park, Uxbridge, Middlesex UB11 1DS, UK	Tel: 01895 251010 Fax: 01895 202999
	1220 Charleston Rd, PO Box 7393, M/S G/11 Mountain View, CA 94039-7393 USA	Tel: 415 969 9112 Fax: 415 964 8331
Advanced Technology Laboratories	Arden Press House, Pixmore Avenue, Letchworth, Herts SG6 1LH, UK	Tel: 01462 679371 Fax: 01462 670899
	OHM Strasse-3, D-85716 Unter Schleissheim, Munich, Germany	Tel: 89 32 17 50 Fax: 89 3173955
	PO Box 3003, Bothell, WA 98041-3003, USA	Tel: 206 487 7000 Fax: 206 487 8100
Aloka (KeyMed in the UK)	6-22-1 Mure, Mitaka-shi, Tokyo 181, Japan	Tel: 0422 45 6049 Fax: 0422 45 4058
BBS Medical Electronic (string phantom) See Seil Imaging in UK	Hagerstensvagen 295, Box 202, S-12902 Hagersten, Sweden	Tel: 468 979 980 Fax: 468 972 004
B & K Medical	Ascot House, Doncastle Rd, Bracknell, Berks RG12 8PE, UK	Tel: 01344 860111 Fax: 01344 860478
Diasonics Sonotron (Vingmed)	2, Napier Road, Bedford MK41 0JW, UK	Tel: 01234 340881 Fax: 01234 266261
	Steinhauserstrasse 74, PO Box 4737 CH-6304 ZUG, Switzerland	Tel: 42 41 6464 Fax: 42 41 6580
	2860 DeLa Cruz Blvd, Santa Clara, CA 95050 USA	Tel: 408 406 4700 Fax: 408 496 3566/ 3561
Dynamic Imaging (only portable systems)	9 Cochrane Square, Brucefield Industrial Park, Livingston EH54 9DR, UK	Tel: 01506 415282 Fax: 01506 410603

Table 2.1. (*cont.*)

Company	Address	Telephone & Fax
Gammex-RMI	34 Shakespeare St, Nottingham NG1 4FQ, UK	Tel: 0115 9483807 Fax: 0115 9484120
	2500 West Beltline Hwy, University Avenue, PO Box 620327 Middleton, WI 53562-0327 USA	Tel: 608 831 1188 Fax: 608 836 9201
GE Medical Systems (Diagnostic Sonar in UK)	Kirkton Campus, Livingston EH54 7BX, UK	Tel: 01506 411877 Fax: 01506 412410
	Paris, France	Fax: 1 40 93 33 33
	Milwaukee, USA	Fax: 1 414 544 3384
Hewlett Packard	Cain Road, Bracknell, Berkshire RG12 1HN, UK	Tel: 01344 369269 Fax: 01344 361051
Key Med	Key Med House, Stock Road, Southend-on-Sea, Essex SS2 5QH, UK	Tel: 01702 616333 Fax: 01702 465677
Kodak (video and printers only)	PO Box 66, Station Rd, Hemel Hempstead, Herts HP1 1JU, UK	Tel: 01442 844480 Fax: 01442 845086
	Eastmann Kodak, 343 State Street, Rochester, New York, NY14650 USA	Tel: 716 724 4000
Kontron	Blackmoor Lane, Croxley Business Park, Watford, Herts WD1 8XQ, UK	Tel: 01923 412214 Fax: 01923 412314
	B.P. 81 F-78185 St Quentin, Yvelines Cedex, France	Tel: 30 57 66 00 Fax: 30 44 23 57
Kretztechnik	Unit 1, Spindle Way, Crawley, Sussex RH10 1TG	Tel: 01293 510231 Fax: 01293 510234
	Tiefenbach 15, A-4871 Zipf, Austria	Tel: 7682 2261-0 Fax: 7682 2261-47

Table 2.1. (*cont.*)

Company	Address	Telephone & Fax
Panasonic (video and printers)	Panasonic House, Willoughby Road, Bracknell, Berks RG12 8FP, UK	Tel: 01344 853205 Fax: 01344 853871
	1, Panasonic Way, Panazip 4B-7 Secaucus, NJ 07094, USA	Tel: 201 392 6091 Fax 201 392 6558
Philips	Kelvin House, 63-75 Glenthorne Rd, Hammersmith, London W6 0LJ, UK	Tel: 0181 741 1666 Fax: 0181 741 7651
	PO Box 10.000 5680 DA Best The Netherlands	Fax: 40 762555
	710 Bridgeport Ave, PO Box 848, Shelton, CT 06484 USA	Tel: 203 926 7674
Pie Medical	Pie Data UK Ltd, Unit 1, Spindle Way, Crawley, West Sussex RH10 1TG, UK	Tel: 01293 510231 Fax: 01293 510234
	Philipsweg 1, 6227 Maastricht The Netherlands	Tel: 43 824600 Fax: 43 824601
	3535 Route 66, Neptune, NJ 07753, USA	Tel: 800 722 6400 Tel: 908 922 4888 Fax: 908 922 3561
Siel Imaging Equipment Ltd (UK distributor for BBS Medical Electronic)	Orpheus House, Calleve park, Aldermaston, Berks RG7 4QW, UK	Tel: 01735 671 828
Siemens	Siemens House, Oldbury, Bracknell, Berks RG12 8FZ, UK	Tel: 01344 396317 Fax: 01344 396337
Sony (video and printers only)	The Heights, Brooklands, Weybridge, Surrey KT13 0XW, UK	Tel: 01932 816000 Fax: 01932 817011

Table 2.1. (*cont.*)

Company	Address	Telephone & Fax
Swift Technologies (Ultrapacs storage only)	Lime Tree Lodge, Church Lane, Owermoigne, Dorchester, Dorset DT2 8HS, UK	Tel: 01305 853782 Fax: 01305 854271
Toshiba	Manor Court, Manor Royal, Crawley, West Sussex RH10 2PY, UK	Tel: 01293 560772 Fax: 01293 560791
	Zilverstraate 1, 2718 RP Zoetermeer, The Netherlands	Tel: 79 689 222 Fax: 79 689 444
	1-1, Shibura 1-Chone, Minoto-KU, Tokyo 1050-01 Japan	Tel: 3 3457 4511 Fax: 3 3456 1631
	82, Totowa Rd, Wayne, NJ 07470, USA	Tel: 201 628 8000 Fax: 201 621 1875
UEEP database (University of Glasgow)	22, Western Court, 100 University Place, Glasgow G12 8SQ, UK	Tel: 0141 211 2953 Fax: 0141 339 1563 Internet:gpinfo@ udcf.gla.ac.uk
VingMed	(see Diasonics Sonotron)	

users in a hospital, and consultation with them may make it possible to negotiate better deals on price and maintenance contracts.

Image storage

The cheapest option for obtaining a hard copy of the video image is to use a thermal printer, which costs around £1000 (at 1995 prices). The paper is also cheap, with each image costing around eight pence. The drawback of this method of image recording is the short life of the image – i.e. five years. Alcohol, if spilt on the images, will rapidly dissolve them, as will sticky tape if used to attach the images to the notes. A less fragile reproduction of the video image, also at low cost, can be made with a thermal transfer printer such as the Sony OP 1200.

Most of the images in this book were made with a video printer that cost £2500 (at 1995 prices). The glossy print produced has a shelf-life of

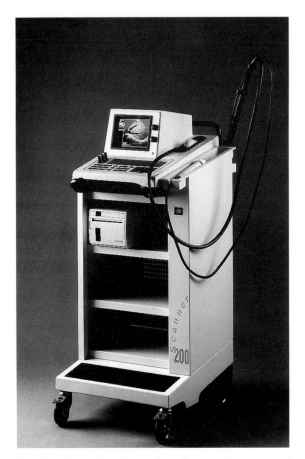

Fig. 2.1. *Example of a small easily portable ultrasound scanner: the Pie Medical 200.*

about 30 years when stored under normal room conditions, but the paper is expensive at around £1 per print. Solvents can damage the records. This type of printer produces a still image from the video screen or playback and will include any colour present on the image. Unfortunately, the frame freeze on most video recorders is not good enough to allow excellent images to be made off-line. Early ultrasound images were photographed from the screen onto Polaroid film but the shelf-life was short, and the method messy and expensive. Any of the other alternatives would be a better current option. Matrix cameras produce X-ray type images which are permanent, but this is a very expensive method of reproduction and at present the films are difficult to store and review easily, although computerised radiology records and filmless departments may improve this.

Picture archiving

Increasingly, picture archiving onto compact or optical disc is developing as the best option. As many as 350–400 pictures with or without colour

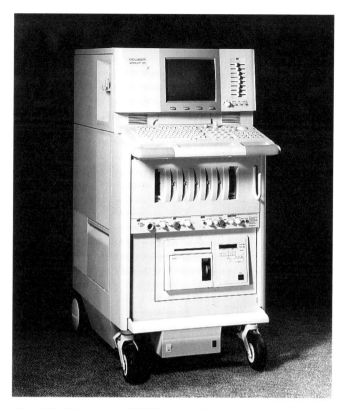

Fig. 2.2. *The Acuson 128XP colour Doppler ultrasound scanner.*

can be stored onto one compact disc ready for rapid retrieval. Personal computer (PC)-based systems are available from Swift Technologies, UK, Ltd, and Acuson have developed a Macintosh-based archiving system. These systems will automatically date and time the picture, they are permanent and can be rapidly retrieved, they occupy very little storage space and are unlikely to become lost. A further advantage is that the pictures can be reviewed on a suitable PC with a compact disc facility without tying up the ultrasound machine for this purpose. New purchasers would be well advised to consider this option seriously.

Video recorders and Doppler signals

Video recording allows movement to be reviewed in real-time and is vital for echocardiography, but less important for other anatomical sites. Doppler signals can be recorded onto the audio channel of the video recorder simultaneously with the image. The quality of this method is usually sufficient to allow off-line calculations for clinical purposes but not good enough for research. Research studies require a more reliable media such as a digital audio tape recorder. Many interested research groups use a PC to acquire the Doppler signal via an interface to the commercial equipment, and if a machine is being purchased with the intention of collecting Doppler signals for research then the type of interface might be of importance. There is always an audio output available, usually via a stereo jack pin meant for headphones, which offers the full Doppler shifted spectrum prior to spectral analysis.

Safe use of ultrasound equipment

Handling babies, their parents and neonatal nurses

Ultrasound is the imaging method of first choice in a neonatal unit because it can be done quickly, safely and repeatedly even with very sick infants. Premature and ill babies are in incubators, often on ventilators and nearly always undergoing monitoring of heart rate, blood pressure, respiration and oxygenation. Intravenous infusions, endotracheal tubes, arterial lines, monitoring probes and feeding tubes are common attachments and the visiting sonographer will become instantly unpopular if he or she inadvertently disconnects any of this equipment. Very ill babies tolerate even gentle handling badly, responding with a falling blood oxygen level. A few moments spent ascertaining how much 'life support' is present and a brief discussion with the baby's nurse regarding the current stability of the patient will pay dividends. Most neonatal units operate an open-door visiting policy so that the baby's parents may be present. An explanation that the technology is the same as that used for antenatal ultrasound and that screening examinations are routine on many neonatal units is usually quickly understood. Parents often wish to remain throughout the procedure and they or their friends may appear through the door of the neonatal unit at any time so that a verbal running commentary is best avoided. The scan pictures and a written explanation should be placed in the notes to be conveyed to the parents via the clinician caring for the baby.

Positioning the baby in the incubator – hats

The baby's head is more likely to remain still if it is turned to one side with his/her body lying prone or supine. Excessive neck twisting should be avoided as venous flow is easily obstructed (Cowan & Thoresen, 1985). Venous obstruction has been implicated in the genesis of intraventricular haemorrhage (Gould *et al.*, 1987). It is usually possible to place the probe on the infant's head without opening the incubator as small probes can be pushed in through the portholes. Some babies are nursed in open cribs (Fig. 2.3a,b). It is important to maintain the infant's temperature during the examination as even the application of cold jelly can contribute to hypothermia which is detrimental. Ultrasound jelly should be kept at room temperature; heating it is not advisable as this can encourage bacterial growth, and also it could easily become too hot.

Endotracheal tube fixation systems vary, the most important point here being that many neonatal units tie the tube, which may be oral or nasal, to a hat (Fig. 2.4a). Check for this before removing the hat. The only way

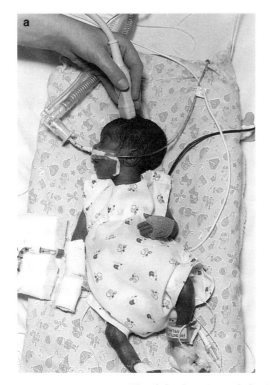 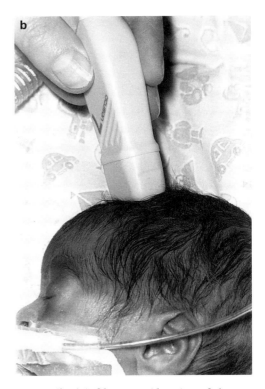

Fig. 2.3. *Imaging a baby in an open crib. (a) Shows a wider view of the scan process. (b) Shows the scan probe in place on the baby's head. Note the operator has her sleeves rolled up and jewellery removed.*

to carry out a cranial ultrasound examination in a baby with this type of tube fixation is to cut a small hole in the hat, which is usually acceptable. Loosening the tape may dislodge the endotracheal tube. Babies may be receiving oxygen piped in via a clear perspex head box in which case it is possible to use a face mask or oxygen tubing instead. This can be held in position for the short time required, although an assistant will be needed. The main obstruction may come from the sticky tape used to fix intravenous lines – sometimes silastic long lines – which originate in the scalp veins. It goes without saying that these must not be removed without permission, and occasionally this will preclude cranial ultrasonography.

Monitoring

Free-breathing, preterm infants are prone to episodes of reduction in heart rate (bradycardia) and brief periods of cessation of breathing (apnoea); hence the widespread use of heart rate and respiratory monitors in neonatal units. Bradycardia is defined as a heart rate of less than 80 beats per minute, and apnoea as 20 seconds cessation of breathing. Oxygen saturation monitors are also commonplace. These are usually set to alarm at below 90% saturation, but frequently give problems because of a poor

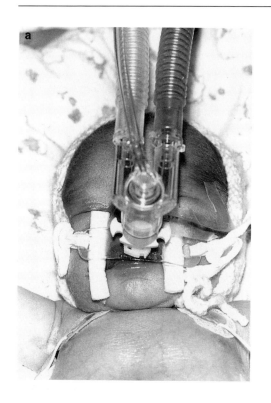
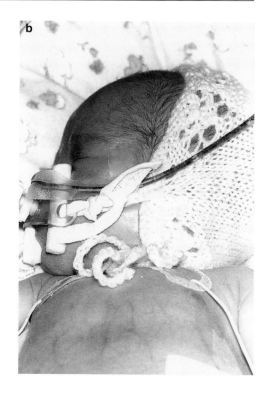
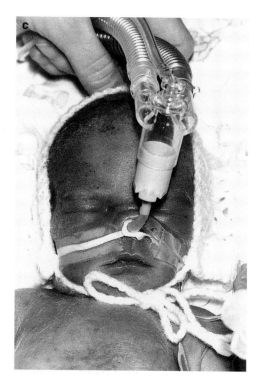
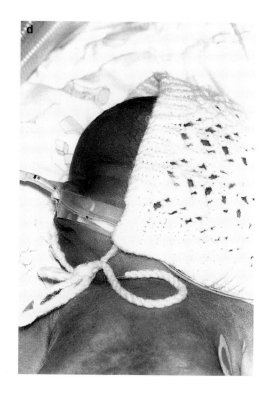

signal from the probe, which is a light source attached to a hand or foot. Alarm limits are set to alert the nursing staff to changes, and nuisance alarms are frequent. If an alarm sounds it is worth checking whether or not it is genuine. Genuine alarms must be acted on and mean that the ultrasound examination should stop until the baby's condition is restored. The baby may be disconnected from the ventilator or have developed a pneumothorax. The increase in intracranial pressure caused by the probe pressing on the fontanelle can cause bradycardia especially in infants with pre-existing intracranial lesions. The vast majority of apnoeic attacks resolve spontaneously or respond to gentle stimulation such as stroking or patting. Reduction in oxygen saturation usually responds to an increase in ambient oxygen and a temporary cessation of the procedure. High blood oxygen levels are also best avoided in view of the association with retinopathy of prematurity and these can result from the use of a face mask in place of a head box during scanning.

Hygiene

Cross-infection is an ever-present risk in a busy neonatal intensive care unit. Newborn babies are poor at fighting infection and ill babies are susceptible because of invasive procedures and indwelling lines. Operators should remove jewellery from the forearms, roll up their sleeves and wash up to the elbows using a chlorhexidine wash followed by an alcohol handrub: Fig. 2.3a represents good practice in this respect. The probe should be wiped with an alcohol soaked swab and then air dried between examinations; the head can be encased in a sterile plastic wrapper or disposable surgical glove. Some probes are sterilisable by immersion in special solution but most are not suitable for immersion in liquid. Ultrasound jelly is not normally a sterile product, although individual sachets of sterile ultrasound jelly can be obtained. I have been unable to find any case reports of cross-infection from shared tubs of jelly, and I currently use a single container which is changed frequently and kept at room temperature.

Acoustic power

The trend towards higher power output from diagnostic ultrasound has now been halted, with manufacturers in the last three years paying more attention to this facet of design. Previously the acoustic power output for imaging sometimes approached levels found only in pulsed Doppler mode. The energy output of equipment is important because of the potential for biological effects as described in Chapter 1. Users should keep up to date with current reports on ultrasound safety and measure the output of their

Fig. 2.4. *Systems of endotracheal tube fixation, (a) and (b) show a Rottenrow endotracheal tube holder fixed to a hat by tapes, (c) and (d) show a nasal endotracheal tube with a tape tied around it taped to the face; the hat is removable.*

31

equipment. The Institute of Physical Sciences in Medicine has published a useful report (Hoskins *et al.*, 1994) on the testing of Doppler ultrasound.

Definition

Acoustic power is defined as the flow of energy across the ultrasound field per unit of time. Power is measured in watts. The intensity refers to the amount of power per unit area in the field, usually square centimetres. For continuous wave ultrasound the intensity measured at the peak is important, and is termed intensity spatial peak (I_{sp}). An average value calculated for the intensity at a specified distance averaged across the field is termed intensity spatial average (I_{sa}). Pulsed ultrasound is intermittent so that energy values are briefly high, and the equivalent measurement is of the intensity spatial peak temporal average (I_{spta}). There are many other measurements of acoustic power, for further information consult the books by McDicken (1991) or Evans *et al.* (1989). A typical value for I_{spta} in B-mode imaging would be 20 mW.cm^{-2}, whereas for PW Doppler the value could easily be 200 mW.cm^{-2}. The range is very wide, and PW units can have energy outputs as high as 4000 mW.cm^{-2}. Rabe *et al.* (1990) measured the power output of several commercial Doppler ultrasound devices that had radiation force balance, used to examine infant brains and found them to vary from 8.7 mW to 96.8 mW. Acoustic pressure is also generated. This can be expressed as the maximum (peak) positive or negative pressure amplitude (p+ and p−). Shock waves can be formed in liquid media when ultrasound passes through so that knowledge of the pressure output may prove particularly important for obstetric users. Although the units of power are in watts, manufacturers commonly label the intensity control in decibels. This is done because of the difficulty of measuring absolute values, which requires a separate calibration for each transducer.

Exposure time

The likelihood of a biological effect depends on the peak energy output and the duration of exposure. The definition of a 'duty cycle' is the ratio of the total on-time to the total examination time. Figure 2.5 plots the relationship between the intensity and the exposure time. The safe zones are derived from knowledge of bio-effects. From the plot it is clear that if the intensity (I_{spta}) is less than 100 mW.cm^{-2} then there is no need to worry about the exposure time. Most machines operate well at this level, but for machines with higher outputs the on-time should be recorded. The American Institute of Ultrasound in Medicine considers that 'there have been no biological effects . . . for unfocused ultrasound below 100 mW.cm^{-2} . . . and even at high intensities when the product of intensity and exposure time is less than 50 joules.cm^{-2}.' One joule per second equals one watt. The British Medical Ultrasound Society also favours a limit of 100 mW.cm^{-2} and proposes a pressure limit of 4 mega pascals.

Measuring power output

The recent international standard IEC 1157 (requirement for the declaration of the acoustic output of medical diagnostic equipment) requires

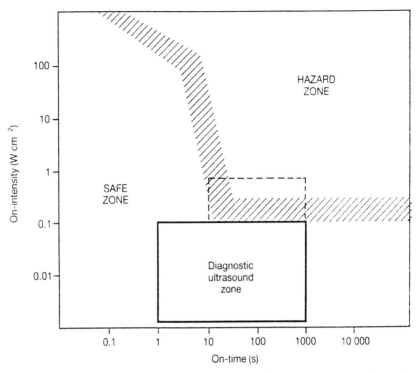

Fig. 2.5. *Relationship between power intensity and exposure time to show safe limits for ultrasound. The box indicated by the dashed line shows the region above 100 mW cm² above which some diagnostic units now fall. (Reproduced with the permission of John Wiley & Sons Ltd; Evans et al., 1989.)*

measurement of the peak negative acoustic pressure and the spatial peak temporal average intensity in a plane which contains the maximum pulse-pressure-squared integral. Power is measured with a radiation pressure balance. These contain a test object which absorbs or reflects ultrasound completely, and thus the object experiences a force due to change in momentum. The force is equivalent to P/c where P is the force and c is the speed of ultrasound: for relecting objects the equation will be 2 P/c. Radiation force balances can measure down to 1±0.1 mW. Measuring such small forces is achieved by placing the absorption material under water on a sensitive chemical balance (Rooney, 1973). Pressure can be measured with a hydrophone containing a tiny piezoelectric crystal. Medical physics departments should be able to assist in checking the power output of ultrasound equipment.

Quality control: accuracy of ultrasound measurements

Quality control has been a neglected area in ultrasound. Considering that important clinical decisions are based on results involving millimetre differences in size of small structures the lack of external standards with

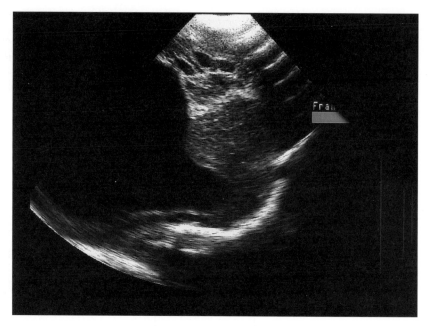

Fig. 2.6. *Ring echoes on the right-hand side of the image caused by a lack of a coupling agent between skin and transducer.*

which to assess the accuracy of the equipment and the operator seems odd. Commercial test objects are available with 'cysts' and wires of differing size embedded in agar gel containing carbon particles, imitating tissue, in which the speed of ultrasound is 1540 m.s^{-1}. Gammex RMI (see Table 2.1 for address) manufacture a suitable grey scale phantom with targets as small as 0.1 mm (model 403GS, in 1995 cost £1443). Repeated use of such test objects allows deterioration in machine performance to be identified. Velocity flow phantoms have been described (Rickey *et al.*, 1992) and are becoming commercially available. Gammex RMI also have a flow phantom available at a cost of £4700 (in 1995) which uses a mixture of glycerol, water and polystyrene microspheres to imitate blood. The very low flow rates of the newborn are difficult to imitate with a phantom: a flow rate of 2 mm.s^{-1} in a 2 mm vessel equals a flow rate of 0.4 ml.min^{-1}. Moving strings of silk or cotton are also used to mimic blood flow (BBS Medical Electronic).

Recognising artefacts

Concentric rings: lack of coupling agent, reverberation echoes

Lack of a coupling agent causes a row of regular echoes to appear resulting from reverberation of ultrasound between the transducer face and the skin (Fig. 2.6). In body structures a similar ring effect can be caused by a

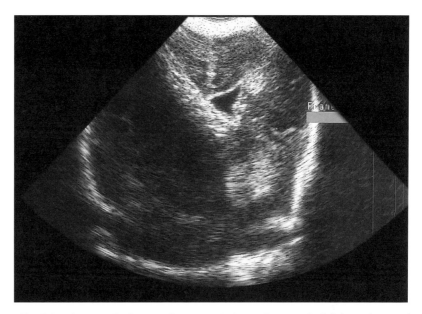

Fig. 2.7. *Acoustic shadow cast by a ventricular catheter in the left lateral ventricle.*

strongly reflecting surface just below and parallel to the transducer. The returned echoes go and return again, thus a reflecting surface becomes apparent at twice the original depth. The artefact may only fade out after several reverberations. Cystic structures containing water or urine are prone to this type of artefact.

Shadowing

A strongly absorbing structure will cast an acoustic shadow behind it; bone and gas are very prone to this. The shadow itself may appear as though it is a small dark echo-transmitting area in contrast to the surrounding tissue and this can be confusing particularly if the tissue has a characteristic speckle pattern which is altered by the presence of the artefact. Figure 2.7 shows an extensive shadow cast by a ventricular catheter.

Mirror image production

The most common example of this is when a second image of liver tissue pattern is seen in the lungs due to the diaphragm acting as a large smooth reflector, but any smooth reflector can act as a mirror scattering ultrasound. Figure 2.8 shows multiple mirror images of a single ventricular catheter.

Noise

Excessive noise and speckle can be produced from incorrect setting of the time-gain compensation control, or introduced by a poor electrical

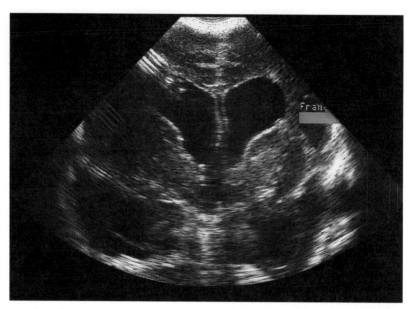

Fig. 2.8. *Mirror images of a single ventricular catheter in the left lateral ventricle.*

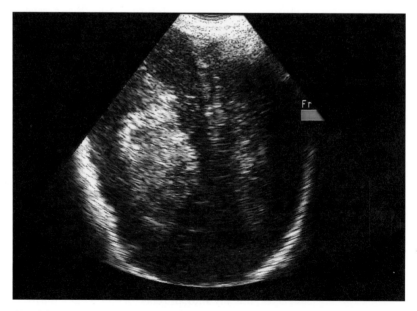

Fig. 2.9. *Excessive speckle in the far field caused by electrical interference.*

connection (Fig. 2.9). Structures beyond liquid containing areas can appear excessively bright compared to neighbouring structures imaged by ultrasound which has not passed through liquid.

References

Cowan, F. & Thoresen, M. (1985) Changes in superior sagittal sinus blood flow velocities due to postural alterations and pressure on the head of the newborn infant. *Pediatrics*, **75**:1038–47.

Evans, D.H., McDicken, W.N., Skidmore, R. & Woodcock, J.P. (1989) *Doppler Ultrasound: Physics, Instrumentation and Clinical Applications*. Chichester: John Wiley & Sons Ltd.

Gould, S.J., Howard, S., Hope, P.L. & Reynolds E.O.R. (1987) Periventricular intraparenchymal cerebral haemorrhage in preterm infants: role of venous infarction. *Journal of Pathology*, **151**:197–202.

Hoskins, P.R., Sherriff, S.B. & Evans, J.A. (1994) *Testing of Doppler Ultrasound Equipment*. Report No. 70. York: Institute of Physical Sciences in Medicine.

McDicken, W.N. (1991) *Diagnostic Ultrasonics*, 3rd edn. Edinburgh: Churchill Livingstone.

Rabe, H., Grohs, B., Schmidt, R.M., Schloo, R., Bömelburg, T. & Jorch, G. (1990) Acoustic power measurements of Doppler ultrasound devices used for perinatal and infant examinations. *Pediatric Radiology*, **20**:277–81.

Rickey, D.W., Rankin, R. & Fenster, A. (1992) A velocity phantom for colour and pulsed Doppler instruments. *Ultrasound in Medicine and Biology*, **18**:479–94.

Rooney, J.A. (1973) Determination of acoustic power outputs in the microwatt-milliwatt range. *Ultrasound in Medicine and Biology*, **1**:13–16.

3 *Normal neonatal cranial ultrasound appearances*

Introduction

The anterior fontanelle provides a convenient acoustic window through which to image the neonatal brain until about one year of age. An infinite number of different images can be produced, but several views have become standard because they allow visualisation of important structures such as the germinal matrix. The pictures and diagrams in this chapter are designed to help the novice ultrasonographer find his or her way around the intracranial anatomical landmarks of these standard views. Once these have been learnt there is then no substitute for time spent trying to identify the same structures in many different subjects. The pathological specimens prepared for this chapter have been cut in the oblique planes which are produced when an ultrasound transducer is angled from the fontanelle. They therefore appear rather different from those in a conventional neuroanatomy book. Useful further information can be obtained from the books edited by Grant (1986) and Richter & Lierse (1991). The pocket ultrasound atlas written by Rumack *et al.* (1990) contains a short, well illustrated section on cranial imaging. All neonatal ultrasound interpretation rests on the initial descriptions by the pioneers Grant *et al.* (1980), Johnson & Rumack, (1980) Slovis & Kuhns (1981) and Shuman *et al.* (1981).

Performing a cranial ultrasound examination

Begin by placing the transducer on the fontanelle with the plane of the ultrasound passing from ear to ear to give a coronal section. The convention is to display the image in the same way as an X-ray, with the left-hand side of the patient on the right-hand side of the image as you look at it on the screen. Set the depth of the image to allow the bright base of the skull to appear at the bottom of the imaged arc, which can be as wide as possible. The depth will correspond to about 7 cm in a small baby. The transducer can then be angled as far forward as the fontanelle will allow, when it is usually possible to identify the orbital ridge of the skull. The transucer is then angled back from this position through at least five 'stations' (Fig. 3.1). When the coronal sections are complete, turn the transducer through 90°, which will place the plane of the image from front to back and produce a parasagittal section. The convention now is to have the baby 'looking' to

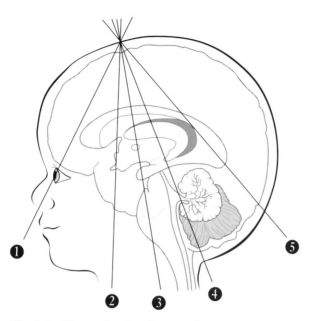

Fig. 3.1. *Planes of section for coronal scans.*

the the left of the picture as shown in the images which follow. The transducer can now be angled to give a plane as near as possible to the surface of the brain, and if the size of the fontanelle allows, an image can be produced which is almost like the external appearance of the whole brain. Several planes of section can be identified including a midline sagittal view (Fig. 3.2).

The whole examination can be recorded on videotape, but if hard copies are required pictures of a coronal section through the region of the third ventricle and an angled parasagittal from both sides are usually made. A detailed examination can be completed in about five minutes with little disturbance to the baby. The examples used in this chapter are from mature infants. The appearance of the very immature brain will be discussed in the next chapter.

Notes on the standard coronal sections

Section 1: frontal lobes (Figs. 3.3 a–d)

The most anterior coronal section contains mostly frontal lobe. The orbital ridge of the skull forms the boundary of this image with a lemon-shaped profile. The grey matter is fairly homogenous but it is often possible to make out a streak of more echodense material which is the anterior limb of the internal capsule. The anterior cerebral arteries can often be seen pulsating as they lie close together in the interhemispheric fissure. Blood vessels provide useful landmarks throughout the examination but their

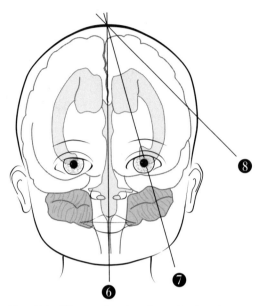

Fig. 3.2. *Planes of section for sagittal and parasagittal scans.*

small size mostly places them below the lower limit of resolution of ultrasound. The base of the skull is consistently the most echo-reflectant structure and provides a basis for comparison of other 'bright' echogenic objects.

Section 2: anterior frontal horns of the lateral ventricles (Figs. 3.4 a–d)

As the transducer is moved in a coronal plane back from the most anterior position the frontal horns of the lateral ventricles appear as slitlike structures just to both sides of the midline. The cerebrospinal fluid within the ventricles transmits ultrasound freely making the cavity appear dark; occasionally the cavity of the ventricle is so small that the walls appear in apposition as bright lines. Mature infants have smaller ventricular cavities than premature infants. In the example the cavity of the left lateral ventricle is almost obliterated. There is often minor asymmetry between the ventricles and this is not pathologic. The cavum septum pellucidum is often very large in preterm babies and lies between the lateral ventricles and not below them, a feature which enables it to be distinguished from the third ventricle. The posterior portion is termed the cavum vergae and this can also be seen in neonatal cranial ultrasound scans. The sulcus of the corpus callosum appears as a bright echo above the cavum with the tissue of the corpus callosum below it.

The other major landmark in this plane during real-time examination comes from the pulsation of the middle cerebral artery arising from the

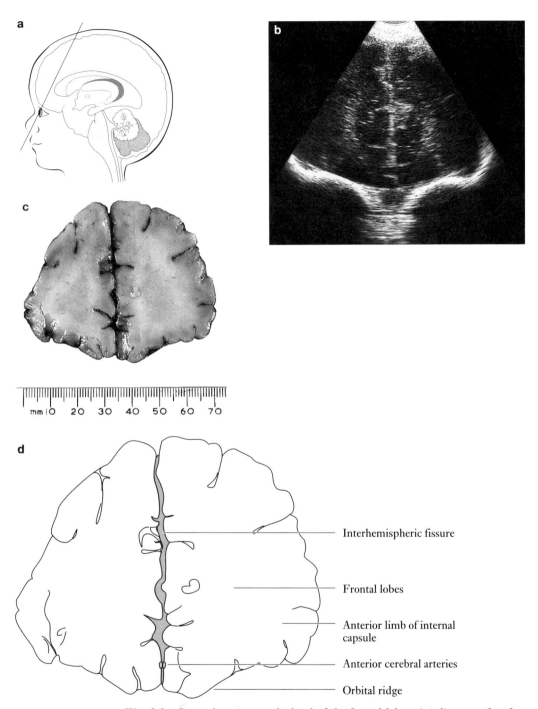

Fig. 3.3. *Coronal sections at the level of the frontal lobes: (a) diagram of surface marking at this level; (b) ultrasound scan corresponding to the plane of section; (c) pathological specimen cut in the plane of section; (d) labelled line diagram to show the main anatomical landmarks.*

41

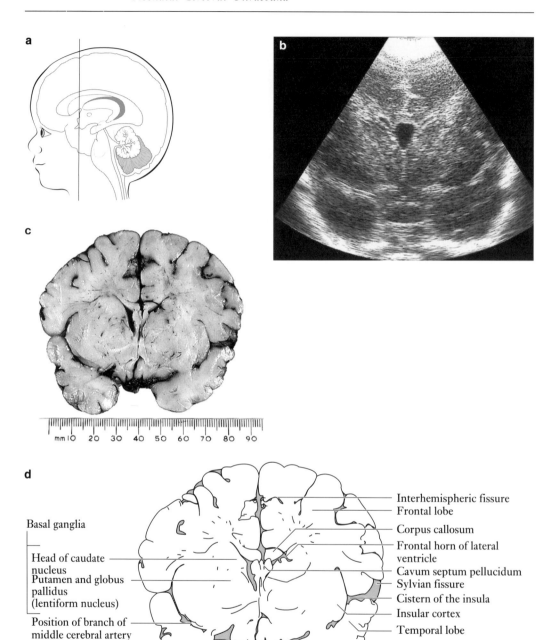

Fig. 3.4. *Coronal sections through the anterior horns of the lateral ventricles: (a) diagram of surface marking at this level; (b) ultrasound scan corresponding to the plane of section; (c) pathological specimen cut in the plane of section; (d) labelled line diagram to show the main anatomical landmarks.*

bifurcation of the internal carotid artery. A long section of the course of the artery can be seen, as in Fig. 3.4 (b), as it travels in the Sylvian fissure demarcating the temporal lobe from the insular cortex on each side. The basal ganglia at this level consist of the caudate nucleus in its position immediately inferior to the lateral ventricles, together with the putamen and the globus pallidus, and these can usually be made out as rather denser appearing grey matter. The boundary in the far field is marked by the 'mask' formed by the sphenoid bone as the transducer is swept from the first to the second station (Cremin *et al.*, 1983).

Section 3: level of the third ventricle (Figs 3.5a–d)

The third ventricle varies considerably in size but can usually be made out as a small echo-free area appearing in the midline, below and between the lateral ventricles and the cavum septum pellucidum. The connections between the lateral and the third ventricle (the foramen of Monro) can be clearly seen on the left side in Fig. 3.5(c). The anatomy of the ventricular system is such an important basis for relating associated structures that a diagram of a cast of the system is given (Fig. 3.6). The pathological specimen (Fig. 3.5c) is at a slightly different level to that of the real-time image (Fig. 3.5b). The image shows the interpeduncular cisterns. The pulsations of the basilar artery can often be seen within the cisterns, which do not appear dark and echo-free like most CSF. The same is true for the quadrigeminal cisterns in the next plane (see Fig. 3.7). The reason for this is thought to be the presence of fine arachnoid trabeculae within these spaces which act as echo-reflectant structures (Mack & Alvord 1982). Throughout these planes of section the Y-shape of the Sylvian fissure provides a constant lateral landmark. This fissure becomes deeper and more convoluted with maturity, as explained in the next chapter. As the plane of the section is moved backwards a fraction these are replaced by the more echodense appearance of the brainstem which appears as a tree or star-like shape. The point at which this becomes very clear marks the transition from the plane of Fig. 3.5 to that of Fig. 3.7.

Section 4: level of the quadrigeminal cisterns (Figs. 3.7 a–d)

The plane of the transducer moves past the brainstem structures, which appear dense, and the bottom midline of the image then contains the cerebellum and the fourth ventricle. The quadrigeminal cisterns appear echo-reflectant, like the interpeduncular cisterns (see above). This prominent appearance has been described as a 'three-pointed crown' (Naidich *et al.*, 1986). The fourth ventricle can sometimes be seen as a relatively echo-free zone above the denser structure of the cerebellar vermis, below which the cisterna magna can be made out far inferiorly in position above the occipital bone of the skull which marks the most inferior part of the image. The cisterna magna is visible in Fig. 3.7(b). The vermis of the cerebellum

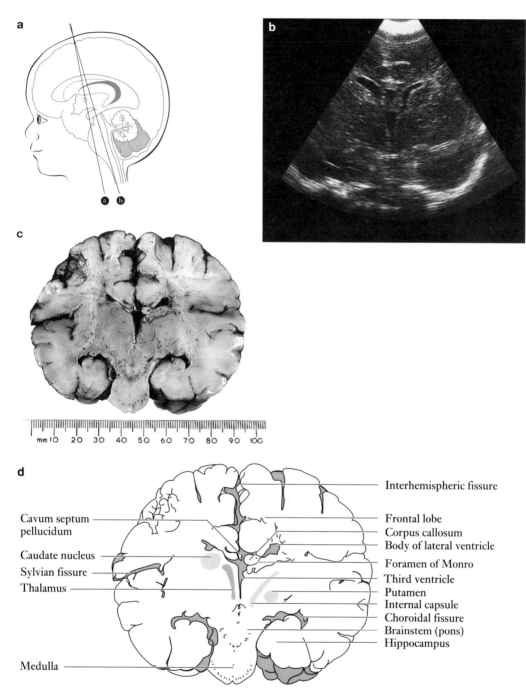

Fig. 3.5. *Coronal sections at the level of the third ventricle: (a) diagram of surface marking at this level – a, plane of scan; b, plane of anatomical section; (b) ultrasound scan corresponding to the plane of section; (c) pathological specimen cut in the plane of section; (d) labelled line diagram to show the main anatomical landmarks.*

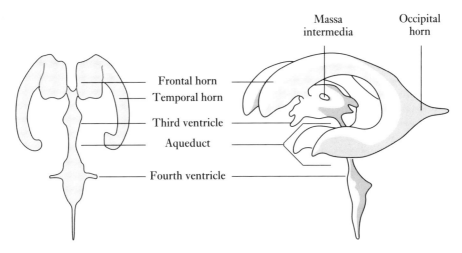

Fig. 3.6. *Diagram of a cast of the ventricular system.*

appears brighter than the cerebellar hemispheres which are bounded by the tentorium cerebelli

The thalamus occupies the position inferior to the bodies of the lateral ventricles. The appearance of the thalamus is usually uniform and relatively hypoechoic, but occasionally bright spots can be identified within it. These have been linked to asphyxia, hyperbilirubinaemia and infection (Weber *et al.*, 1992). Examples are given in Chapters 9 and 11. The ultrasound scan shown in Fig. 3.7(b) is symmetrical and relates more to the left-hand side of the pathological specimen (Fig. 3.7d) which has been cut rather obliquely.

Section 5: level of the trigone (Figs. 3.8 a–d)

Scanning further posteriorly gives a tangential cut through the trigone of the lateral ventricles, which dominates the most posterior sections. The glomus of the choroid plexus fills the cavity of the lateral ventricles in this position, and is particularly large in preterm babies. Choroid plexus haemorrhage can be difficult to diagnose and depends on asymmetry of the appearances. Choroid plexus cysts are a common finding during pregnancy and have been reported in as many as 3% of newborns (Riebel *et al.*, 1992). In this plane the white matter around the ventricles tends to appear quite echodense. This appearance has been termed the 'peritrigonal blush' (Di Pietro *et al.*, 1986) or 'periventricular halo' (Grant *et al.*, 1983). This appearance has been described in full-term neonates (Laub & Ingrisch, 1986). The blush is thought to be due to the neurovascular bundles travelling at right angles to the ultrasound beam and thus acting as a good reflector, as in premature babies they are surrounded by a brain with a high water content. Myelin was not present in this region at postmortem in 28 preterm cases (Di Pietro *et al.*, 1986). Normally the blush

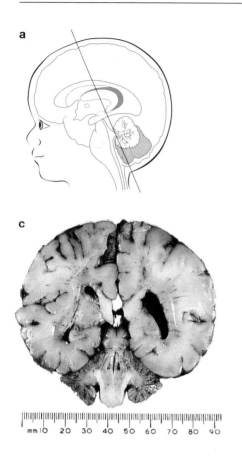

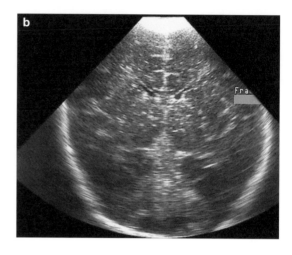

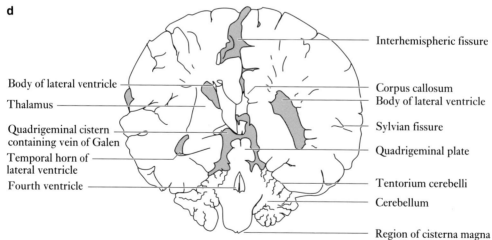

Body of lateral ventricle

Thalamus

Quadrigeminal cistern
containing vein of Galen

Temporal horn of
lateral ventricle

Fourth ventricle

Interhemispheric fissure

Corpus callosum
Body of lateral ventricle

Sylvian fissure

Quadrigeminal plate

Tentorium cerebelli

Cerebellum

Region of cisterna magna

Fig. 3.7. *Coronal sections at the level of the quadrigeminal cisterns: (a) diagram of surface marking at this level; (b) ultrasound scan corresponding to the plane of section; (c) pathological specimen cut in the plane of section; (d) labelled line diagram to show the main anatomical landmarks.*

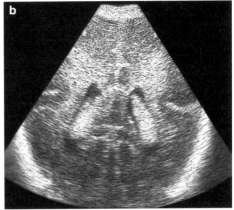

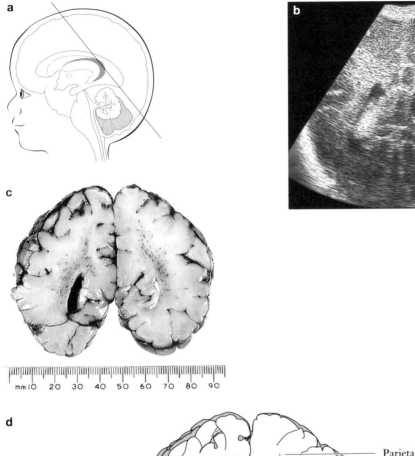

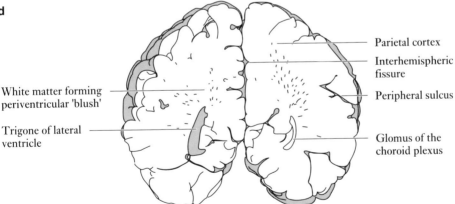

White matter forming
periventricular 'blush'

Trigone of lateral
ventricle

Parietal cortex

Interhemispheric
fissure

Peripheral sulcus

Glomus of the
choroid plexus

Fig. 3.8. *Coronal sections at the level of the trigone: (a) diagram of surface marking at this level; (b) ultrasound scan corresponding to the plane of section; (c) pathological specimen cut in the plane of section; (d) labelled line diagram to show the main anatomical landmarks.*

is less bright than the skull base or the choroid plexus and is symmetrical, with the appearance of fine brush strokes. The normal range of appearance is of importance as there is a need to distinguish between blush and a 'flare' in this region which may represent subtle pre-white matter injury, perhaps resulting from inflammatory cell infiltrate. Persistent flare has been correlated with abnormal neurodevelopmental outcome (see Chapter 12). The cavum vergae can sometimes be seen between the lateral ventricles in this view.

By angling the transducer even further posteriorly, the occipital cortex can be imaged. This is a useful plane for confirming the presence of flare and for looking for the small occipital cysts of periventricular leukomalacia.

Section 6: midline sagittal (Figs. 3.9 a–d)

This useful image gives a great deal of information. In the midline, the cerebellar vermis forms a highly echogenic landmark in the posterior fossa, with its anterior surface dented by a small cleft which is the fourth ventricle. The surface area of the cerebellum seen in this view has been estimated, and correlated well with the post-conceptional age (Birnholz, 1982). The pons is anterior to this and is not particularly echogenic. Inferior to the cerebellum is the echo-free zone of the cisterna magna. Arising from the superior surface of this structure and extending upwards is the echogenic quadrigeminal cistern which formed an important landmark in the coronal section 4 (Fig. 3.7). Pulsations of the basilar artery can be recognised within this cistern during a real-time examination. This bright band terminates in a tongue of choroid plexus in the roof of the third ventricle (the tela choroidea). Anterior to this is the third ventricle itself, which is a rhomboidal shape bounded by the 'figure of three' effect generated by its choroid. The inferior boundary of the third ventricle is formed by the interpeduncular cistern which also appears bright like the quadrigeminal cistern. The massa intermedia can be made out only when hydrocephalus is present.

The corpus callosum can be seen sweeping from the anterior to posterior direction in the midline view, with the superior cingulate sulcus above and parallel to it. The parieto-occipital sulcus forms another clear landmark above the posterior fossa. In mature infants the sulci are more branched than in immature infants, and the superior cingulate sulcus itself is more developed posteriorly.

Section 7: angled parasagittal (Figs. 3.10 a–d)

This section is dominated by the 'C' shape of the lateral ventricle. This is variable in size, tending to be smaller in term infants. The caudate nucleus lies below the floor of the frontal horn of the lateral ventricle with the thalamus behind and below it. The caudate nucleus is usually more echogenic than the thalamus. The glomus of the choroid plexus fills the occipital horn of the lateral ventricle. The choroid plexus tucks in the caudothalamic

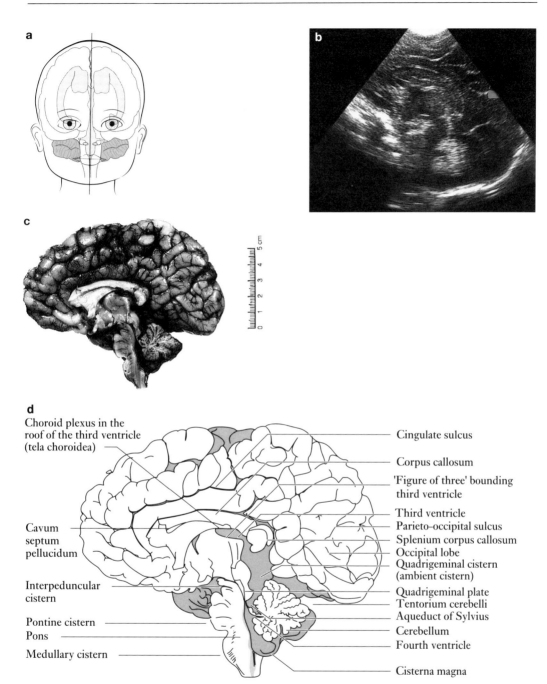

a

b

c

d

Choroid plexus in the
roof of the third ventricle
(tela choroidea)

Cavum
septum
pellucidum

Interpeduncular
cistern

Pontine cistern
Pons

Medullary cistern

Cingulate sulcus

Corpus callosum

'Figure of three' bounding
third ventricle

Third ventricle
Parieto–occipital sulcus
Splenium corpus callosum
Occipital lobe
Quadrigeminal cistern
(ambient cistern)

Quadrigeminal plate
Tentorium cerebelli
Aqueduct of Sylvius
Cerebellum
Fourth ventricle

Cisterna magna

Fig. 3.9. *Midline sagittal sections: (a) diagram of surface marking at this level; (b) ultrasound scan corresponding to the plane of section; (c) pathological specimen cut in the plane of section; (d) labelled line diagram to show the main anatomical landmarks.*

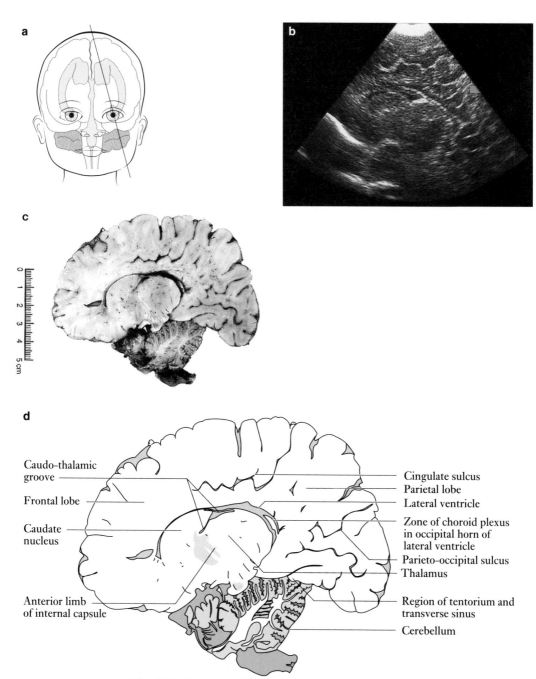

Fig. 3.10. *Parasagittal sections through the lateral ventricles: (a) diagram of surface marking at this level; (b) ultrasound scan corresponding to the plane of section; (c) pathological specimen cut in the plane of section; (d) labelled line diagram to show the main anatomical landmarks.*

groove in the floor of the lateral ventricle and often forms a bright spot, as in the example. This is normal and should not be confused with a small haemorrhage into the germinal matrix capillary bed which is situated over the head of the caudate in a slightly more anterior position.

Section 8: tangential parasagittal (Figs. 3.11 a–d)

Further lateral angulation of the scanhead will produce a section which is tangential and superficial to the lateral ventricle. The Sylvian fissure is the landmark in this view. The number of sulci which can be identified increases with maturity. In less mature infants the insula can be glimpsed, as the opercula have not yet fully enclosed it.

Axial section at the level of the cerebral peduncles

An axial section can be made by placing the transducer on the scalp above the relatively thin temporal bone. This view does not employ the anterior fontanelle as a window. This section corresponds to that obtained in conventional CT imaging.

Normal variation

Cavum septum pellucidum and cavum vergae

The large size of the cavum septum pellucidum is often a striking feature in cranial ultrasound images of preterm babies. The structure varies in size from a cavity much larger than that of the adjacent ventricles (Fig. 3.12) to a small slit (Fig. 3.13). The cavum septum pellucidum has disappeared by two months of age in 85% of cases (Shaw & Alvord, 1969). Closure of the cavum vergae begins at about 24 weeks of gestation. The cavum septum pellucidum can enlarge to a pathologic cyst (Garza-Mercado, 1981), and haemorrhage into it has been described (Butt *et al.*, 1985). The width of the cavum septum pellucidum varied from 2 mm to 10 mm in 102 preterm infants studied by Ferrugia & Babcock (1981). The cavi are often in communication with each other but not with the ventricular system.

Cerebrospinal fluid spaces

The lateral ventricles often differ considerably in volume, particularly in the occipital horns. For detail about the normal range of linear and area measurements see Chapter 9. The cisterna magna can be difficult to visualise and can also vary in height, the mean value being 4.5 mm (Goodwin & Quisling, 1983). Small size of the cisterna magna can be a clue to the presence of the Arnold-Chiari malformation. The subarachnoid spaces are more prominent in very preterm babies, with the appearance of separation of the Sylvian and interhemispheric fissures. Measurement of the

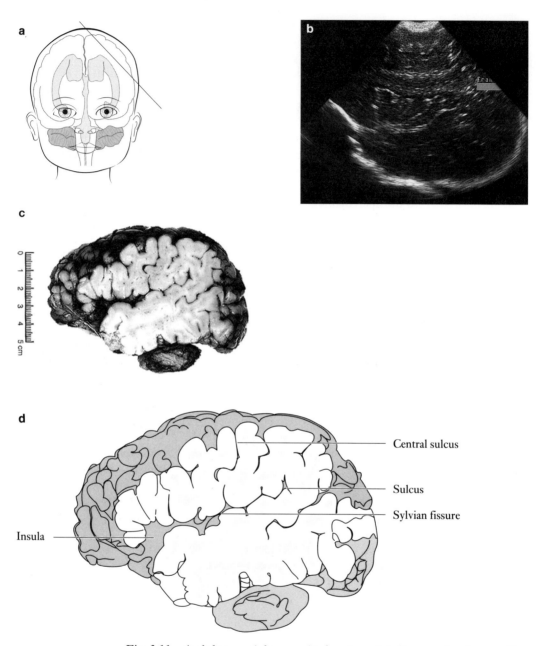

Fig. 3.11. *Angled tangential parasagittal sections: (a) diagram of surface marking at this level; (b) ultrasound scan corresponding to the plane of section; (c) pathological specimen cut in the plane of section; (d) labelled line diagram to show the main anatomical landmarks.*

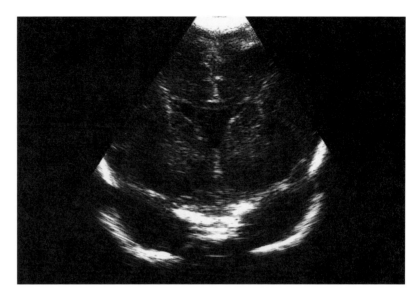

Fig. 3.12. *Coronal section showing large cavum septum pellucidum.*

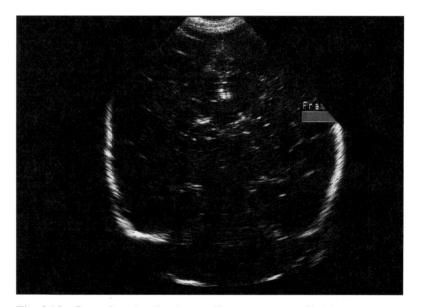

Fig. 3.13. *Coronal section showing small cavum septum pellucidum.*

subarachnoid space using a 10 MHz transducer was reported by Govaert *et al.* (1989) in a section similar to that in Fig. 3.14. The results showed dimensions of less than 5 mm in normal newborns, similar to those obtained using magnetic resonance imaging in 48 newborns (McArdle *et al.*, 1987). The subarachnoid space was often particularly wide over the parieto–occipital lobes. An isolated finding of a widened subarachnoid

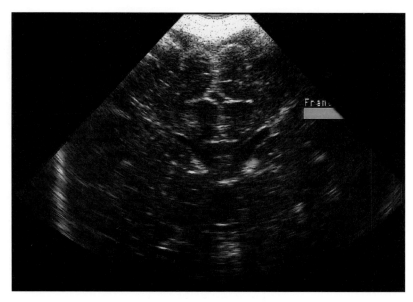

Fig. 3.14. *Coronal section showing the subarachnoid space at the top of the picture, close to the transducer.*

space (no measurements were given) was reported in six of a cohort of 75 preterm Canadian infants (Lui *et al.*, 1990), all of whom developed normally.

References

Birnholz, J.C. (1982) Newborn cerebellar size. *Pediatrics*, **70**:284–7.

Butt, W., Havill, D., Daneman, A. & Pape, K. (1985) Haemorrhage and cyst development in the cavum septi pellucidi and cavum vergae. *Pediatric Radiology*, **15**:368–71.

Cremin, B.J., Chilton, S.J. & Peacock, W.J. (1983) Anatomical landmarks in anterior fontanelle ultrasonography. *British Journal of Radiology*, **56**:517–26.

Di Pietro, M.A., Brody, B.A. & Teele, R.L., (1986) Peritrigonal echogenic 'blush' on cranial sonography: pathologic correlates. *American Journal of Radiology*, **146**: 1067–71.

Ferrugia, S. & Babcock, D.S. (1981) The cavum septi pellucidi: its appearance and incidence with cranial ultrasonography in infancy. *Radiology*, **139**:147–50.

Garza-Mercado, R. (1981) Giant cyst of the septum pellucidum. *Journal of Neurosurgery*. **55**:646–50.

Goodwin, L. & Quisling, R. (1983) The neonatal cisterna magna: ultrasonic evaluation. *Radiology*, **149**:691–5.

Govaert, P., Pauwels, W., Vanhaesbrouck, P., De Praeter, C. & Afschrift, M. (1989) Ultrasound measurement of the subarachnoid space in infants. *European Journal of Pediatrics*, **148**:412–3.

Grant, E., Schellinger, D., Borts, F., McCullough, D., Friedman, G., Sivasubramanian, K. & Smith, Y. (1980) Real time sonography of the neonatal and infant head. *American Journal of Neuroradiology*, 1:487–92.

Grant, E., Schellinger, D., Richardson, J., Coffey, M. & Smirniotopoulous, J. (1983) Echogenic periventricular halo: normal sonographic finding or neonatal cerebral haemorrhage. *American Journal of Neuroradiology*, 4:43–6.

Grant, E.G. (1986) *Neurosonography of the Preterm Neonate*. New York, Springrt-Verlag.

Johnson, M. & Rumack, C. (1980) Ultrasonic evaluation of the neonatal brain. *Radiologic Clinics of North America*, 18:117–31.

Laub, M.C. & Ingrisch, H. (1986) Increased periventricular echogenicity (periventricular halos) in neonatal brain: a sonographic study. *Neuropaediatrics*, 17:39–43.

Lui, K., Boag, G., Daneman, A., Costello, S., Kirpalani, H. & Whyte, H (1990) Widened subarachnoid space in pre-discharge cranial ultrasound: evidence of cerebral atrophy in immature infants? *Developmental Medicine and Child Neurology*, 32:882–7.

McArdle, C.B., Richardson, C.J., Nicholas, D.A., Mirfakhraee, M., Hayden, C.K. & Amparo, E.G. (1987) Developmental features of the neonatal brain: MR imaging. *Radiology*, 162: 230–4.

Mack, L. & Alvord, E. (1982) Neonatal cranial ultrasound: normal appearances. *Seminars in Ultrasound*, 3:216–30.

Naidich, T.P., Yousefzadeh, D.K. & Gusnard, D.A. (1986) Sonography of the normal neonatal head. II. Supratentorial structures: state of the art imaging. *Neuroradiology*, 28: 408–27.

Richter, E. & Lierse, W. (Translated by A. E. Oestreich) (1991) *Imaging Anatomy of the Newborn*. Baltimore: Urban & Shwarzenberg.

Riebel, T., Nasir, R. & Weber, K. (1992) Choroid plexus cysts: a normal finding on ultrasound. *Pediatric Radiology*, 22:410–12.

Rumack, C.M., Horgan, J.G., Hay, T.C. & Kindsfater, D. (1990) *Pocket Atlas of Pediatric Ultrasound*. New York: Raven Press.

Shaw, C.M. & Alvord, E.C., Jr. (1969) Cava septi pellucidi et vergae: their normal and pathological states. *Brain*, 92:213–14.

Shuman, W., Rogers, J., Mack, L., Alvord, E. & Christie, D. (1981) Real-time sonographic sector scanning of the neonatal cranium: technique and normal anatomy. *American Journal of Neuroradiology*, 2:349–56.

Slovis, T. & Kuhns, L. (1981) Real time sonography of the brain through the anterior fontanelle. *American Journal of Radiology*, 136:277–86.

Weber, K., Riebel, Th. & Nasir, R. (1992) Hyperechoic lesions in the basal ganglia: an incidental sonographic findings in neonates and infants. *Pediatric Radiology*, 22:182–6.

4 *The immature brain*

Introduction

The stage of development of the cerebral fissures, sulci and gyri can give an indication of the degree of maturity of the brain. A gyrus is bounded by two sulci or one sulcus and one fissure. The most important landmarks are the parieto-occipital sulcus, the lateral sulcus (Sylvian fissure) and the cingulate sulcus (Fig. 4.1). Chi *et al.* (1977) made a detailed study of 507 brains that were between 10 and 44 weeks gestation, and documented the appearance and development of the major sulci and gyri. The ultrasound appearances lag behind the anatomical description because the sulci have to be quite well-defined before they are detected with ultrasound. The appearances seen in very preterm babies born at around 22–23 weeks gestation are those of a smooth brain surface with few sulci and gyri. The parieto-occipital fissure forms a deep groove on the midline surface of the brain but the insula is wide open and the island of Reil clearly visible in the tangential view. On coronal section, the Sylvian fissure thus appears wide open. Scoring systems have been devised for the ultrasound appearances of immature brains in standard sections (Murphy *et al.*, 1989), or comparison can be made with published photographs such as those in this chapter or in the literature (Fig. 4.2 reproduced from Dorovini-Zis & Dolman, 1977). Details of the scoring system are given in Figs. 4.3 to 4.5, although the standard deviation was wide (Fig. 4.6) meaning that the method has not proved accurate enough for clinical practice. Others have measured the height of the frontal lobes with ultrasound as an index of brain growth and maturity but this was not more sensitive than head circumference (Battisti *et al.*, 1986). The following description of the landmarks is summarised from the published studies (Worthen *et al.*, 1986; Murphy *et al.*, 1989; Slagle *et al.*, 1989; Huang, 1991). Maturation proceeds independently of gestational age at birth unless there is brain injury when it can be retarded (Slagle *et al.*, 1989).

Gestation: 23–24 weeks (Figs. 4.7a–e)

The brain is virtually completely smooth with a wide Sylvian fissure and a large cerebrospinal fluid space between the interhemispheric fissure seen in coronal section. The cingulate sulcus is not yet obvious. The tangential and midline views are dominated by the Y-shaped appearance of the parieto-occipital fissure which has a short stem to the Y at this stage.

56

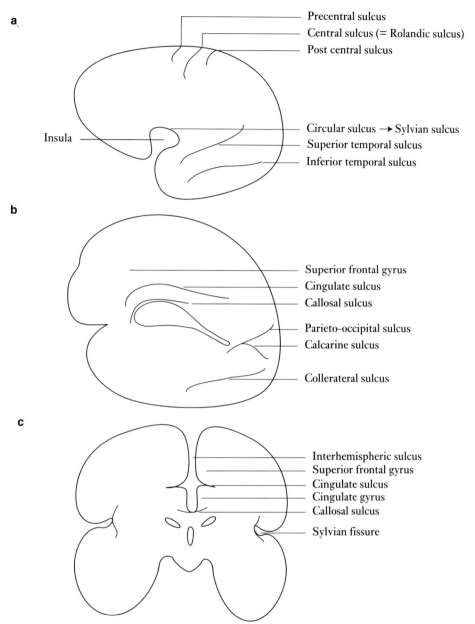

Fig. 4.1. *The major features of the brain which change during maturation: (a) tangential view; (b) midline and parasagittal views; (c) coronal view.*

Gestation: 25–26 weeks (Figs. 4.8a–e)

The edges of the Sylvian fissure have just come together but this is not yet branched, and the cingulate sulcus can usually be seen in the anterior portion in the midline or parasagittal view by 26 weeks, although it is not

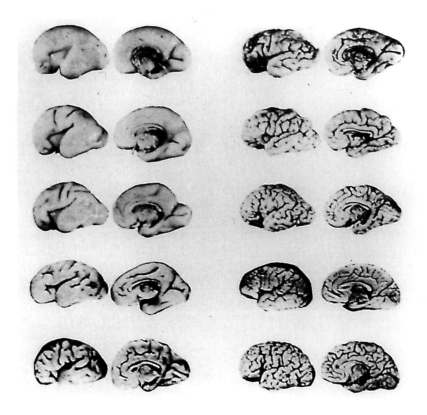

Fig. 4.2. *Characteristic configuration of fetal brain from 22 to 40 weeks of gestation at two-week intervals. All the brains have been brought to the same size. (Reproduced from Dorovini-Zis & Dolman, 1977.)*

yet continuous. The calcarine fissure branches from the parieto-occipital fissure giving a long stemmed Y shape. The frontal and parietal sulci are appearing as dimples.

Gestation 27–28 weeks (Figs. 4.9a–e)

The Sylvian fissure is deepening but the insula is still partly uncovered. The cingulate sulcus is now complete and straight, stretching almost front-to back but there are no secondary branches yet. The parieto-occipital fissure is still clearly seen and some occipital gyri have developed. The post-Rolandic fissure is present. The superior temporal sulcus is present.

Gestation 29–31 weeks (Figs. 4.10a–e)

The Sylvian fissure is now quite deep, completely covering the insula, and the cingulate sulcus quite obvious in the coronal section. The cinglate

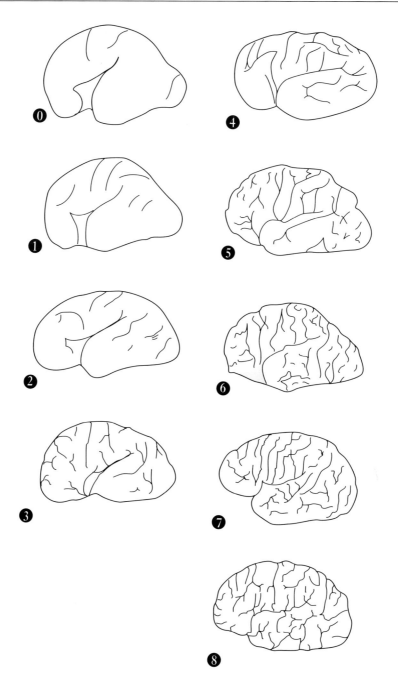

Fig. 4.3. *Scoring system for the appearance of the brain in tangential section.*

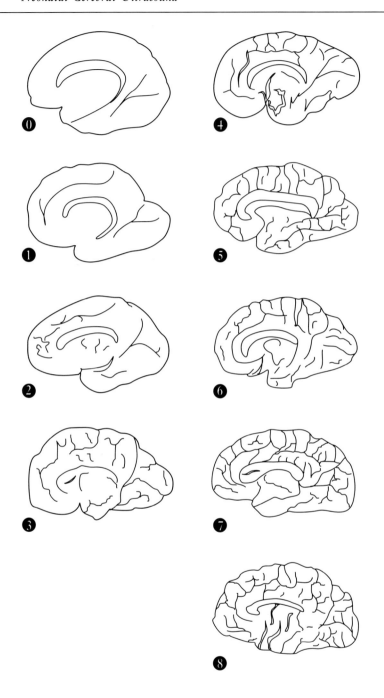

Fig. 4.4. *Scoring system for the appearance of the brain in the parasagittal and midline view.*

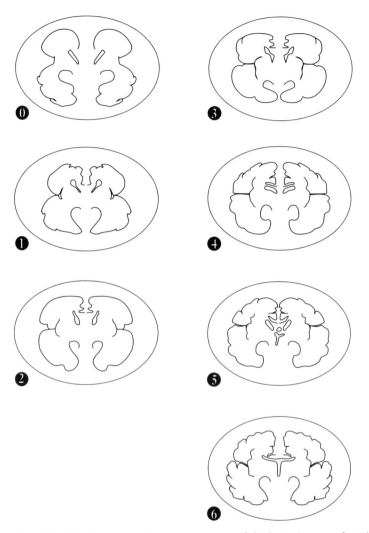

Fig. 4.5. *Scoring system for the appearance of the brain in coronal section.*

sulcus is now curvy and secondary branches can be seen. The parieto-occipital fissure is becoming slightly tortuous in the midline and tangential sections. The inferior temporal sulcus appears by 30–31 weeks whereas it is not present at 28–29 weeks. It can be seen below the Y-shaped parieto-occipital and calcarine fissure in the ultrasound scan example.

Gestation: 32–33 weeks (Figs. 4.11a–e)

Secondary gyri are becoming apparent branching from the superior frontal, parietal and temporal gyri, increasing the complexity of the ultrasound appearances. Insular sulci start to develop making the peripheral Y shape

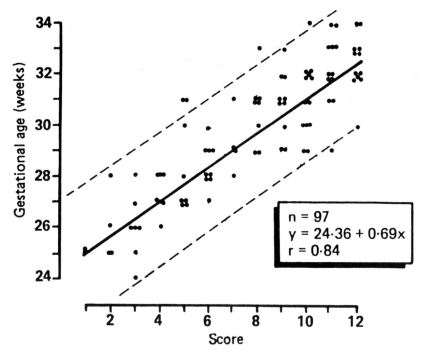

Fig. 4.6. *Relationship of the total score of the brain, estimated from the appearances in Figs. 4.3 to 4.5 to the gestational age. (Reproduced with permission of BMJ Publications from Murphy et al., 1989.)*

of the Sylvian fissure, seen in the coronal sections, a deeper and more complex structure.

Gestation: 35–36 weeks (Figs. 4.12a–e)

This period is characterised by a continuing increase in complexity of the sulci and gyri. Secondary gyri are now obvious in all the coronal and parasaggital sections.

Gestation: 37–42 :term (Figs. 4.13a–e)

Tertiary sulci are present making the superficial appearances resemble a bag of worms, very different to the featureless appearances of the 23-week gestation infant. The cingulate sulcus is extensive and branched, with many minor gyri apparent. This appearance has been described as 'cobblestone' (Slagle *et al.*, 1989). All the sulci and gyri seen in adult brains can now be recognised and after this time brain maturation is characterised by increasing complexity rather than the development of new sulci and gyri.

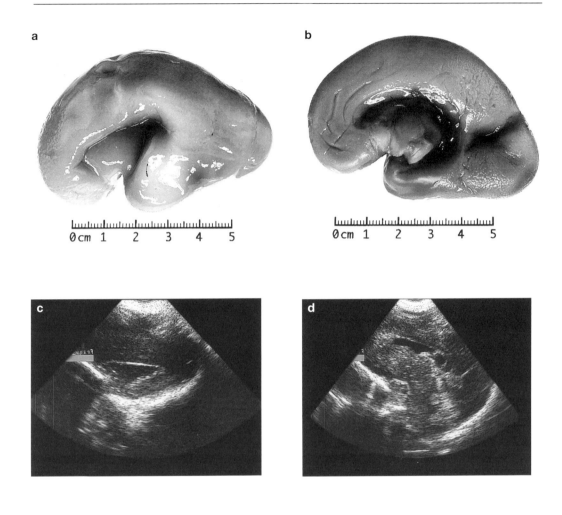

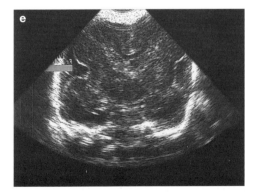

Fig. 4.7. *Appearance of the brain at post-mortem and on ultrasound at 24 weeks' gestation: (a) the superficial appearance of the brain; (b) the midline cut surface; (c) a tangential view; (d) a midline view; (e) a coronal section.*

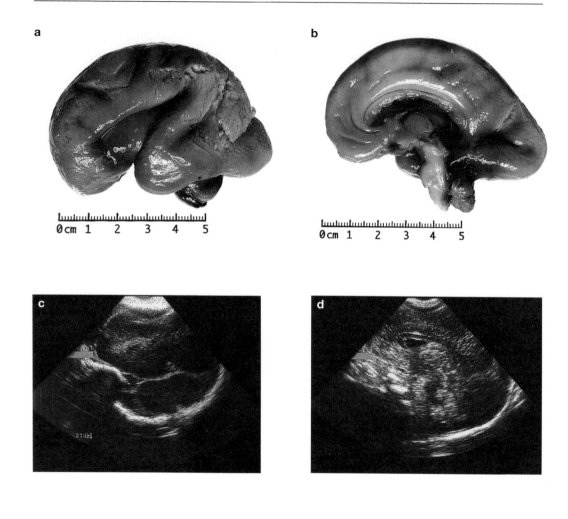

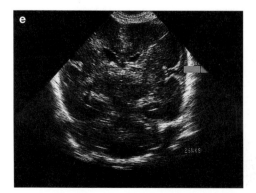

Fig. 4.8. *Appearance of the brain at post-mortem and on ultrasound at 26 weeks' gestation: (a) the superficial appearance of the brain; (b) the midline cut surface; (c) a tangential view; (d) a midline view; (e) a coronal section.*

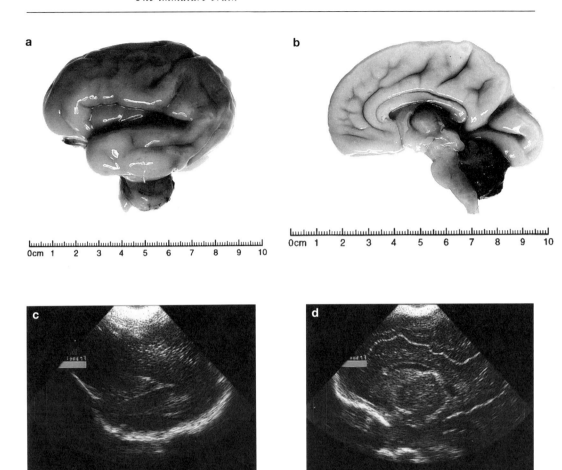

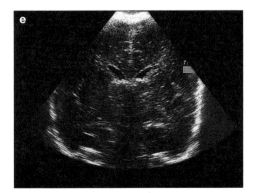

Fig. 4.9. *Appearance of the brain at post-mortem and on ultrasound at 28 weeks' gestation: (a) the superficial appearance of the brain; (b) the midline cut surface; (c) a tangential view; (d) a midline view; (e) a coronal section.*

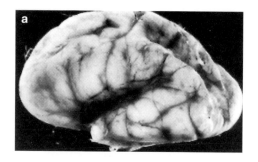
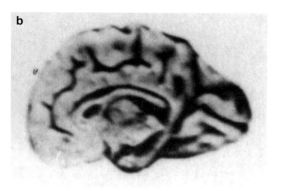
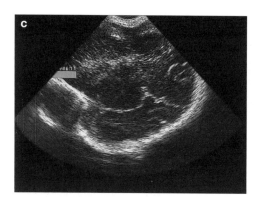
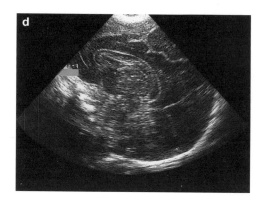
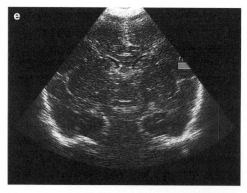

Fig. 4.10. *Appearance of the brain at post-mortem and on ultrasound at 30–31 weeks' gestation: (a) the superficial appearance of the brain (from Pape & Wigglesworth, 1979); (b) the midline cut surface (from Dorovini-Zis & Dolman, 1977); (c) a tangential view; (d) a midline view; (e) a coronal section.*

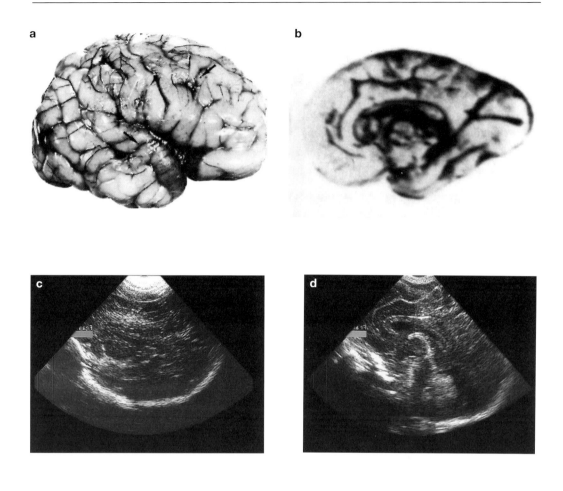

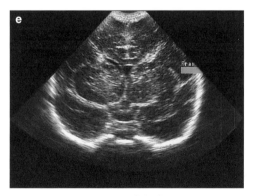

Fig. 4.11. *Appearance of the brain at post-mortem and on ultrasound at 33 weeks' gestation: (a) the superficial appearance of the brain (from Pape & Wigglesworth, 1979), (b) the midline cut surface (from Dorovini-Zis & Dolman, 1977); (c) a tangential view; (d) a midline view; (e) a coronal section.*

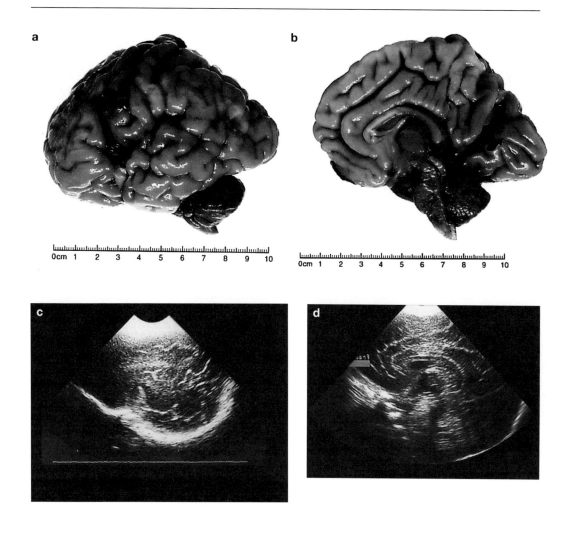

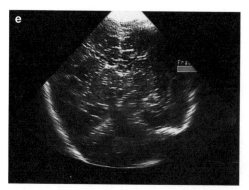

Fig. 4.12. *Appearance of the brain at post-mortem and on ultrasound at 35 weeks' gestation: (a) the superficial appearance of the brain; (b) the midline cut surface; (c) a tangential view; (d) a midline view; (e) a coronal section.*

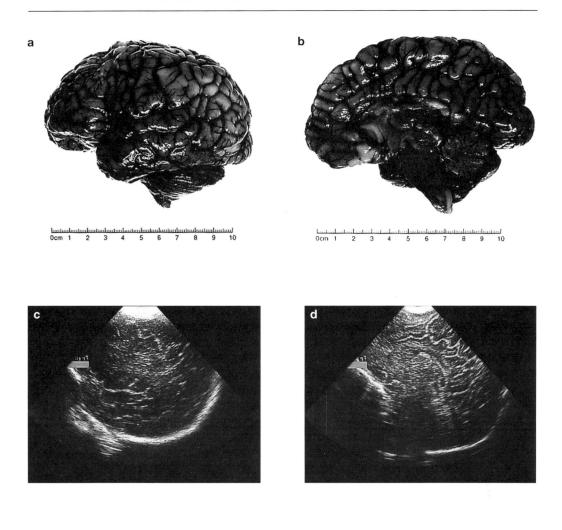

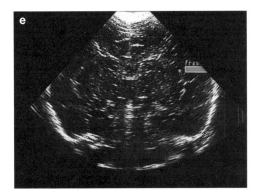

Fig. 4.13. *Appearance of the brain at post-mortem and on ultrasound at term: (a) the superficial appearance of the brain; (b) the midline cut surface; (c) a tangential view; (d) a midline view; (e) a coronal section.*

69

Hypoechoic rims developing around the major sulci at term have also been described and interpreted as representing myelination (Farrell & Birnholz, 1987).

References

Battisti, O., Bach, A. & Gerard, P. (1986) Brain growth in sick newborn infants: a clinical and real-time ultrasound analysis. *Early Human Development*, 13:13–20.

Chi, J.G., Dooling, E.C. & Gilles, F.H., (1977) Gyral development of the human brain. *Annals of Neurology*, 1:86–93.

Dorovini-Zis, K. & Dolman, C.L. (1977) Gestational development of the brain. *Archives of Pathology and Laboratory Medicine.* 101:192–5.

Farrell, E.E. & Birnholz, J.C. (1987) Neonatal neurosonography. *Pediatrics*, 79: 1044–8.

Huang, C.-C. (1991) Sonographic cerebral sulcal development in premature newborns. *Brain Development*, 13:27–31.

Murphy, N.P., Rennie, J.M. & Cooke, R.W.I. (1989) Cranial ultrasound assessment of gestational age in low birthweight infants. *Archives of Disease in Childhood*, 64:569–72.

Pape, K.E. & Wigglesworth, J.S. (1979). *Haemorrhage, Ischaemia and the Perinatal Brain. Clinics in Developmental Medicine*, Nos. 69/70. London: Spastics International Medical Publications.

Slagle, T.A., Oliphant, M. & Gross, S.J. (1989) Cingulate sulcus development in preterm infants. *Pediatric Research*, 26:598–602.

Worthen. N.J., Gilbertson, V. & Lau, C. (1986) Cortical sulcal development seen on sonography: relationship to gestational parameters. *Journal of Ultrasound in Medicine*, 5:153–6.

5 *Monitoring the neonatal brain using Doppler ultrasound*

The anatomy of neonatal cerebral arteries

The anterior cerebral artery can be seen pulsating in a parasagittal image of the brain as it courses around the anterior part of the lateral ventricle and divides into the pericallosal and marginal artery. Identification of the course of the artery is made easier with the addition of colour Doppler (Plate 5.1 and Fig. 5.1). In the first description of the technique a continuous wave ultrasound pencil probe was placed on the anterior fontanelle and angled towards the face. The probe was assumed to be detecting flow in the pericallosal branch of the anterior cerebral artery as it curved around the genu of the corpus callosum, thus travelling directly towards the probe and making an angle correction unnecessary (Bada *et al.*, 1979). A good signal can be obtained from the ascending portion of the anterior cerebral artery midway between its origin from the anterior communicating artery and the inferior portion of the corpus callosum (Plate 5.1). Signals can be obtained from the middle cerebral artery (MCA) through the temporal bone (Plate 5.2 and Fig. 5.2) in a manner similar to that described in adults and older children (Aaslid *et al.*, 1982; Kirham *et al.*, 1986). The whole circle of Willis has been interrogated from this position (Raju *et al.*, 1989; Wong *et al.*, 1989). The anatomical relationships of the middle cerebral artery allow a transducer to be fixed to the head for semi-continuous monitoring (Fig. 5.3).

Obtaining a good Doppler signal

Once a cerebral artery has been identified it is an apparently simple matter to switch into Doppler mode and obtain a signal. Before using the result for research or to aid a clinical decision the best possible signal must be obtained. Most equipment offers the range of frequencies as an audio signal. The human ear is extremely sensitive and it is worthwhile always listening to Doppler output as well as looking at the sonogram. Both these modalities help the operator to make the minor adjustments which are necessary to obtain the best transducer position. Duplex Doppler equipment enables the angle of insonation to be kept as low as possible and measured if necessary, and helps to assess whether any venous flow is

71

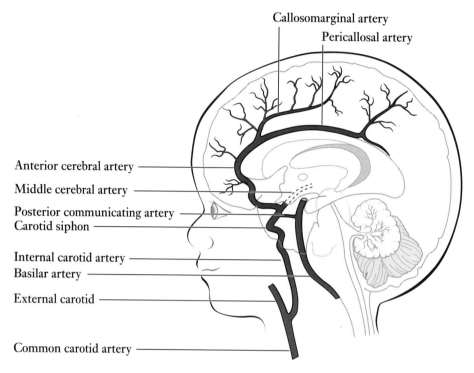

Callosomarginal artery
Pericallosal artery

Anterior cerebral artery

Middle cerebral artery

Posterior communicating artery
Carotid siphon

Internal carotid artery
Basilar artery

External carotid

Common carotid artery

Fig. 5.1. *Anatomical diagram of the course of the artery.*

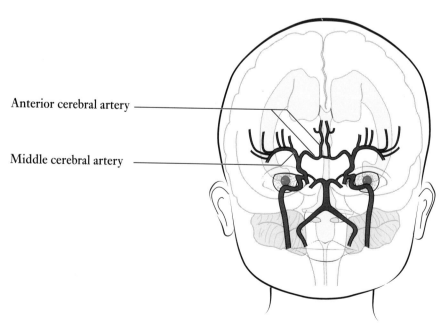

Anterior cerebral artery

Middle cerebral artery

Fig. 5.2. *Anatomical drawing to show the vascular landmarks of Plate 5.2.*

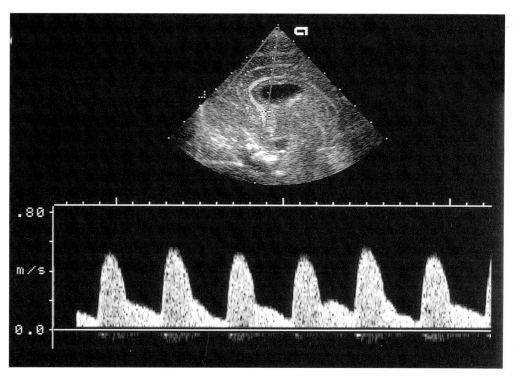

Plate 5.1 *Colour Doppler identification of the anterior cerebral artery.*

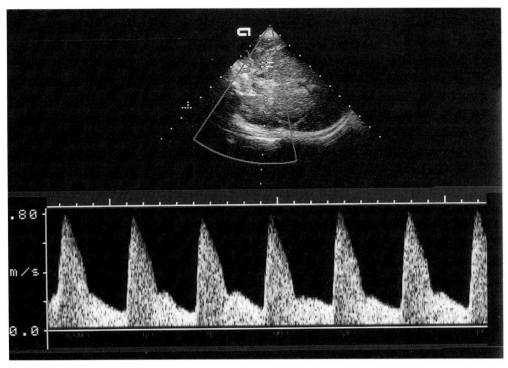

Plate 5.2 *Colour Doppler identification of the middle cerebral artery*

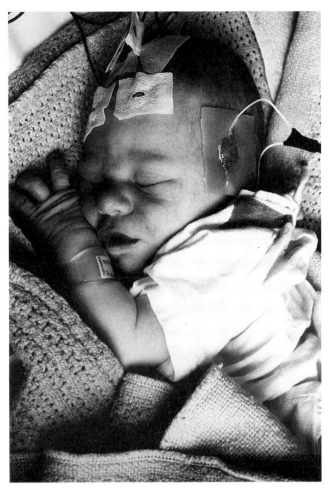

Fig. 5.3. *Transducer fixed on skin of temporal bone of skull for semi-continuous monitoring.*

crossing the path of the beam. Continuous wave (CW) Doppler has a low power output making it more suitable for continuous monitoring. The power of CW output is less than 50 mW.cm^{-2}, compared to 100 mW.cm^{-2} for duplex and colour systems. Neonatal cerebral arteries are uniformly small and the range-gate on duplex equipment should be set to a sample size of 3 mm or less; the transducer beam width is large enough to encompass the vessel. The sample is actually a tear drop shape in three dimensions. Commercial equipment is fitted with a 'wall-thump' filter to remove low frequencies and this should be set to the lowest possible setting, usually 100 Hz. Even this setting results in a gap between the baseline and the bottom of the sonogram which can be a problem at low velocities. Figure 5.4 shows a sonogram obtained from a baby with a large patent ductus arteriosus in which velocity is generally very low. There is missing

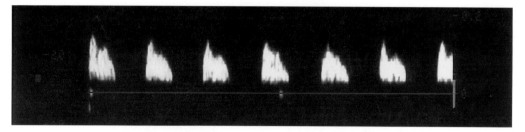

Fig. 5.4. *Low velocity flow in the anterior cerebral artery – the problem of the low-pass filter.*

information at the slowest velocities meaning that it is impossible to tell if there is low-velocity flow present in the reverse channel, as might be expected. The gain may need to be high to detect such low velocities and this can result in the introduction of background noise. Whilst it may be possible to supress this by ear during observation at the cot-side, a noisy signal can be a problem if it is recorded for later automatic signal processing. Aliasing (Chapter 1) is not usually of concern in the neonatal cerebral circulation, but if it is suspected a check should be made with CW Doppler.

Analysis of neonatal Doppler information

Spectral analysis

The returning Doppler shifted spectrum which has insonated a blood vessel contains a wealth of complex information. Blood flowing within the vessel is travelling at different velocities at different times in the cardiac cycle and at different places within the vessel cavity. The frequency components need to be analysed, the best method being that of Fourier transform spectral analysis. The results are displayed as a visual sonogram. The spectral analyser takes in 5 msec of complex signal, resolving the frequencies within it and displaying the result as an array of pixels (spots on a television-type screen). The length of each pixel represents 5 msec and the height is usually one-hundredth of the total frequency range. The grey scale which is assigned to each pixel is a measure of the power of the frequency componenet of that pixel (Fig. 5.5). When looking at a sonogram one can assess the shape, which is usually pulsatile with a shoulder on the downstroke. The sonograms may or may not be regular in shape and size across the recording. The maximum velocity in systole and disastole can be assessed from the scale on the Y axis and the display adjusted accordingly. There may be lack of flow or reversed flow in diastole (Fig. 5.6). The sonogram may be filled in by spectral broadening or may have a clear window beneath the maximum velocity. Further measurements such as the maximum velocity, or the time-averaged mean velocity can be made from the frozen screen display or from the output recorded on audio tape.

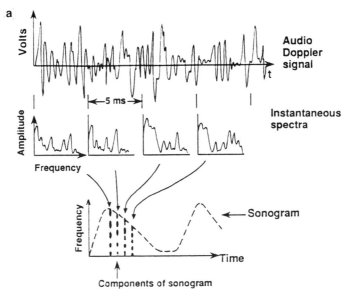

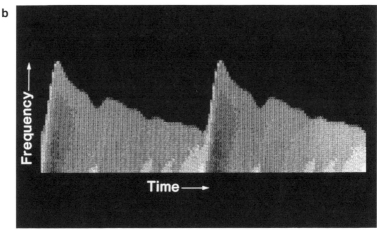

Fig. 5.5(a) and (b). *The build-up of a sonogram. (Reproduced with permission from Churchill Livingstone; McDicken, 1991.)*

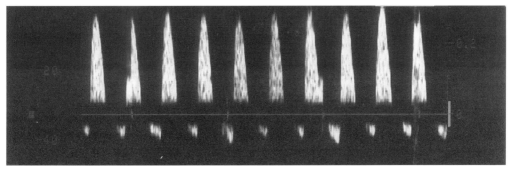

Fig. 5.6. *Example of reversed diastolic flow in patent ductus arteriosus.*

75

Recording Doppler signals

There is a large amount of information contained in a Doppler signal, and it is common to make recordings for later off-line analysis. A picture of the sonogram can be made on Polaroid film or using a video thermal imager. The velocity and time scales should be optimised to show the fine detail, and the sensitivity set to present the sonogram to show some speckle inside the envelope. Audio tape recorders allow prolonged recordings to be made and are convenient for preserving information in a form that can be subjected to further analysis. Forward and reverse channels can be recorded on stereo equipment. *Digital* audio tape recorders have a superior performance but are relatively expensive.

Mean velocity calculations

Plug flow occurs when virtually all the blood is travelling at the same velocity and the Doppler sonogram is empty beneath the maximum velocity components (this is also referred to as lack of spectral broadening). The sonogram from the arteries of the neonatal brain does not assume plug flow characteristics and flow is probably laminar, or occurring in concentric rings of different velocities with the slowest next to the arterial wall. Due to small size the whole of the vessel is insonated with the Doppler beam, thus the sample represents the full range of velocities within the vessel. The best estimate of the mean velocity of flow over the whole cardiac cycle is obtained by tracing the peak velocity envelope, integrating the frequencies over time, calculating the mean velocity from the Doppler equation given in Chapter 1 and then halving it (Evans, 1985). This method does not rely on uniform insonation of the vessel, which is required if the mean velocity envelope is used instead of the peak envelope. Unfortunately there is no agreement on which is the best method. The neonatal Doppler literature reports normal ranges calculated from maxiumum and minimum velocities, time-averaged mean velocity from the peak envelope and the intensity-weighted mean velocity both halved and not (Table 5.1).

Waveform indices

Various mathematical indices can be derived from the sonogram and if they involve ratios of velocities they have the attraction of being angle-independent. This is because the cosine factor in the Doppler equation appears in the numerator and denominator and hence cancels out. The resistance index of Pourcelot is often reported in the neonatal literature and referred to as PI.

$$PI = \frac{\text{Peak systolic velocity} - \text{end diastolic velocity}}{\text{Peak systolic velocity}}$$

Table 5.1. *Published normal Doppler cerebral blood flow velocity values in term and preterm neonates*

Reference	N	Subjects	Equipment	Artery	Results + comments
Ando et al. (1983)	43	normal term	Parks CW	ACA	velocity increase over first few days, PI decreased
Gray et al. (1983)	23	normal term	5 MHz Medasonics CW special	ACA in three places	PI reducing over first 3 days – about 0.75. Upslope and downslope angle analyses
Archer et al. (1985)	24	normal term	4 MHz CW with spectral analysis	ACA in three places	PI reduces over first 5 days – about 0.7
Ando et al. (1985)	35	<37 weeks, 14 normal, 13 RDS, 8 SEH	Parks CW	ACA	PI reduced in norms, more variable in SEH, higher in IVH group – 0.8 to 0.6
Drayton & Skidmore (1987)	10 30	term preterm <33wk	ATL Mk 600 with offline analysis	ACA, MCA	velocity increase in first 72 hours. Term 7.5 cm.sec^{-1}, preterm 4.5 cm.sec^{-1} MCA>ACA
Raju et al. (1987)	19 6	term stable preterm	ATL Mk 500 duplex	common carotid	term peak velocity about 54 cm.sec^{-1}, mean 33: preterm 47,41
Raju & Zikos (1987)	22 25	term preterm	HP phased array Duplex pulsed 5 MHz	ACA, different sites	Area under curve 4–7 waveforms peak 15 cm.sec^{-1} reduced by 40% from ICA to pericallosal
Sonesson et al. (1987)	20	normal term	Vingmed 2 MHz range-gated	Internal carotid	reduction in first 30 min then no change in mean first 3 days though change in syst and diast
Shuto et al. (1987)	91	stable term	Toshiba pulsed duplex 5 MHz	ACA & basilar	PI only reported; correlation with GA; 0.9 preterm 0.6 term
Mirro & Gonzalez (1987)	25	normal term perinatal	5 MHZ CW Medasonics	?ACA	PI 0.75 before birth, 0.53 after birth

Table 5.1. (*cont.*)

Reference	N	Subjects	Equipment	Artery	Results + comments
Bode & Wais (1988)	25 112	newborn older child	EME 2 MHz pulse with FFT	MCA, ACA	increase over 20 days, mean 25–45 cm.sec⁻¹, peak 45–75 cm.sec⁻¹
Strassburg et al. (1988)	20	normal term	CW 4 and 8 MHz zero crossing	ACA common carotid	velocity increase first 72 hours, peak syst 35–55 cm.sec⁻¹, PI 0.7 to 0.5
Calvert et al. (1988)	29	ventilated <32 weeks	Medasonics CW 8MHz	ACA	increase mainly first 16 hr value about 2: fall in PI
Evans et al. (1988)	27	<1500g	ATL Mk 600 5 MHz	ACA, MCA	mean velocity 4.5 cm.sec⁻¹ ACA, 6.5 MCA; PI 0.8; inc. first 3 days. Resistance area product (BP/CBFV) fell
Ramaekers et al. (1989)	8	preterm 26–32 weeks	CW 2 MHz Doptek	ACA	PI correlated with heart rate, more variable active sleep
Deeg & Rupprecht (1989)	121	29–45 weeks	Acuson 128 colour + PW	ACA, B + ICA	velocity higher in ICA and related to gestational age
Jorch et al. (1990a)	12	31–40 weeks	ATL Mk 500	ACA	mean 10 cm.sec⁻¹ PI 0.8 (0.56–0.92)
Fenton et al. (1990)	128	normal term	ATL Mk 600 offline analysis	MCA, ACA	increase first 72 hours esp first 24; 8 cm.sec⁻ ACA, (6–10), 12 cm.sec⁻ MCA (8–12); PI 0.7 (0.6–0.8)
Lui et al. (1990a)	10 10	term preterm	ATL Mk 450	ACA, MCA	PI only reported
Winberg et al. (1990)	20	preterm <34 weeks	Vingmed 5 MHz	Int carotid	reduction first 5 hours then increase. Mean about 12 cm.sec⁻¹

Reference	N	Population	Equipment	Vessels	Findings
Van de Bor & Walther (1991a)	83	normal term	ATL UM8 duplex, 5 MHz	ICA, basilar, ACA	pericallosal branch ACA peak 28 cm.sec^{-1}, mean 15 cm.sec^{-1}; PI 0.79. No correlation PI with vel
Kurmanavichius et al. (1991)	17	<1500g	Acuson 128 colour 3.5 MHz, Doptek offline	MCA	increase in mean vel due to increased diastolic; 13 cm. sec^{-1} to 17.5 in 12 hours.
Yoshida et al. (1991)	69	mixed: about 16 in each group	EME TC2 2 MHz	MCA	increase mainly first few days: mean velocity about 18 cm.sec^{-1}
Hayashi et al. (1992a)	40	normal term	Aloka 550350 duplex	ACA, internal carotoid	peak ACA 35 cm. sec^{-1}, decrease 0–3 hours then increase
Connors et al. (1992)	16	normal term	ATL UM9 colour duplex	Internal carotid, basilar	PI reduced 8 hours after birth compared to prenatal
Mires et al. (1994)	217	normal preterms <37 weeks	HP5 MHz Duplex	MCA, ACA	RI fell first 12 hours (0.75 range 0.65–0.83); higher in <33 week infants than more mature during first 12 hours only
Cheung et al. (1994)	50	mixed including SGA	Aloka 5 MHz Dupex	ACA	PI reduced, lower in SGA infants in first 24 hours

RDS; respiratory distress syndrome; HP; Hewlett Packard; UM: commercial abbreviation; SEH: subependymal haemorrhage; FFT: fast Fourier transform; RI: resistance index; ACA: anterior cerebral arteries; MCA: middle cerebral artery; IVH: intraventricular haemorrhage; CW: continuous wave; ICA: internal carotid artery; PI: Pourcelot index; SGA: small for gestitional age; BP: blood pressure; ATL: Advanced Technology Laboratories; PW: pulsed wave; CBFV: cerebral blood flow velocity; EME: electro medical engineering.

If the resistance to flow is low, the value of the ratio is low since there is high flow in diastole. Pourcelot's index should be differentiated from the pulsatility index of Gosling – often also abbreviated to PI in the adult literature – which is the peak systolic velocity minus the end diastolic velocity divided by the mean of the maximum velocity. Many other ratios and angles have been described but none have become so widely used as the PI (Gray *et al.*, 1983).

Sources of error

There are many potential sources of error in the calculation of neonatal cerebral blood flow velocity (CBFV). The method suffers from the major drawback that the diameter of any neonatal cerebral artery is below the lower limit of resolution of ultrasound imaging so that quantitative flow can never be estimated. Changes of velocity over time can therefore result from a change in blood flow or change in vessel diameter. Errors arise from non-uniform insonation, and from inaccuracy in estimation of the angle of insonation when this is required. A 3° error in angle measurement at around 40° introduces an error of ±5%. This error is not systematic, and is the reason for avoiding angle corrections in velocity estimations whenever possible. Further errors are introduced by the fact that there is often plane misalignment between the imaging and the Doppler transducers. The velocity may be turbulent not laminar thus complicating the process of calculating the average velocity. The sample of velocities is obtained in a teardrop shape rather than in a cylinder fashion and the velocity of ultrasound in blood is actually 1580 cm.sec^{-1}, not 1540 which is the value ascribed by most manufacturers. These errors, if applied to a poorly obtained and badly recorded sonogram, can make the whole process of estimating velocity meaningless.

Normal values

From published reports several conclusions can be made about neonatal Doppler studies. The arterial velocities are low when compared with adult values, of the order of 8 cm.sec^{-1} (Table 5.1). Cerebral blood flow (CBF) is known to be low in the newborn of most species and the few absolute figures available suggest values of around 11 ml.100 g brain weight.min^{-1} for the human neonate (Volpe *et al.*, 1983; Greisen *et al.*, 1984). Cerebral blood flow velocity values are about 15% lower in premature babies than those born at term. All the published reports suggest an increase of velocity and a reduction of PI during the first few days of life. Several observers have made recordings very early in life and these show an initial reduction in velocity in preterm but not term infants before the gradual increase begins (Sonesson *et al.*, 1987; Winberg *et al.*, 1990; Lui *et al.*, 1990a) although the latest report (Hayashi *et al.*, 1992b) also described an initial reduction in velocity for term infants. Sleep state can affect CBFV; Ramaekers *et al.* (1989), Jorch *et al.* (1990a) Fischer *et al.* (1991) and Ferrarri *et al.* (1994) have studied CBFV in quiet and active sleep. Mirro & Gonzalez (1987), Meerman *et al.* (1990) and Connors *et al.* (1992) report changes just before and after birth. All suggest a reduction after delivery compared to prenatal life, and Meerman's results support the general finding of a relationship between CBFV and gestational age as the velocity steadily increased during fetal life. Table 5.1 also shows how varied the reported 'normal' range is. Some of this variation arises from the use of different equipment, different methods of analysis and reporting, and the fact that the measurements are made in many different branches of the arterial tree. On the whole the more proximal the artery, the higher the velocity. No standard method for performing neonatal Doppler studies has been agreed, and most of the results are based on small numbers of cardiac cycles which may not represent the average velocity over longer periods because of the presence of cycling (Anthony *et al.*, 1991; Coughtrey *et al.*, 1992). The inter-observer variation can be as low as 5% (Lui *et al.*, 1990a) or as high as 15% (Winberg *et al.*, 1986). Kempley & Gamsu (1993a) reported the intra-observer variability as 10%. These high figures must include an effect from physiological cycling. There are two large studies of normal term infants (Fenton *et al.*, 1990, Van de Bor & Walther, 1991a). The largest study of 217 preterm infants reported only the resistance index (Mires *et al.*, 1994). Only Drayton & Skidmore (1987) and Raju & Zikos (1987) have attempted quantitiative estimation of CBF, using a subtraction method across the thoracic aorta and volumetric flow from the carotid artery.

Venous velocities have been described using colour ultrasound to identify the straight section of the vein of Galen. The range was from 5.6 to 13 cm.sec^{-1} in the study of Winkler & Helmke (1989) and 2.3 to 9.5 cm.sec^{-1} in that of Fenton *et al.* (1991).

Validation studies

There have been few attempts at validation between measures of velocity and flow in neonatal animal models. There was poor agreement between hydrogen clearance estimation of flow (Fick principle) in an appropriate area of cortex and Doppler estimate of velocity of the middle cerebral artery in adult cats or neonatal piglets (Morris *et al.*, 1989; Rennie *et al.*, 1990). In piglets which were only a few hours old the CBF was more sensitive to changes in blood pressure than change in arterial carbon dioxide tension (Rennie *et al.*, 1990), and this has been confirmed by others (Haaland *et al.*, 1995). Change in blood pressure also confounded the results of Fenton *et al.* (1992) in preterm human newborns, and this feature of newborn mammals makes many of the validation studies difficult to interpret. Good correlations were obtained between changes recorded with an electromagnetic flowmeter on the common carotid artery and Doppler velocity estimates in piglets only during a narrow range of blood pressure and carbon dioxide changes (Haaland *et al.*, 1994; Thoresen *et al.*, 1994). Reasonable correlations were obtained in adult dogs (Guldvog *et al.*, 1980) and puppies (Raju *et al.*, 1987). The Doppler velocity recorded from the anterior cerebral artery correlated better than PI with changes in CBF measured using microspheres in newborn dogs (Batton *et al.*, 1983). Thoresen *et al.* (1994) found that changes were underestimated by Doppler ultrasound when they were induced by transfusion of incompatible or overheated blood, and the same was true at extremes of blood pressure suggesting that some vasoconstriction may have occurred. Poor results were obtained comparing MCA velocity against xenon measurements of CBF in adult patients with cerebrovascular disease, although there was excellent agreement between the two methods when the percentage change induced by change in carbon dioxide tension was compared rather than the absolute value (Bishop *et al.*, 1986). Changes in CBF induced by changes in carbon dioxide in human newborns have shown a larger percentage change for CBFV measured with Doppler than the change in total CBF recorded using radioactive xenon: 44% per kPa versus 11% per kPa with xenon (Archer *et al.*, 1986a; Greisen & Trojaborg, 1987). In newborn lambs the change in velocity was 2% per mmHg change in carbon dioxide estimated with Doppler compared to a 3.8% change in blood flow measured with microspheres (Sonesson & Herin 1988). Busija *et al.* (1981) observed the pial artery through an operating microscope and recorded a change from 388 μm to 450 μm in hypercapnia. That changes associated with hypercapnia appear to take place at the level of the pial vessels, which can oscillate in synchrony with ventilation, was also suggested by Auer & Sayama (1983). Table 5.2 shows a summary of some of the published validation studies.

Information from clinical Doppler studies in the newborn

Physiological changes

Carbon dioxide

Doppler CBFV studies during changes in carbon dioxide tension have been performed mainly as an indirect validation of the method, and indeed changes in CBFV have been shown to occur with the same magnitude and in the same direction as change in CBF. Carbon dioxide has a potent effect on CBF which doubles after an increase from 40 mmHg to 80 mmHg in healthy adults (Harper & Glass, 1965). Doppler studies in adults showed a change of similar magnitude in CBFV with a median reactivity of around 25% per kPa rise in carbon dioxide tension (Hague *et al.*, 1980; Markwalder *et al.*, 1984). A reduction in PI was shown in 11 healthy full term babies who rebreathed for five minutes (Archer *et al.*, 1986a). This was mainly due to a rise in diastolic velocity which was thought to indicate cerebral vasodilatation, and the result was confirmed in preterm infants by Van Bel *et al.* (1988a), with an additive effect of an associated hypoxia. In a further study of 19 ventilated preterm babies, a rise of 1 kPa in arterial carbon dioxide was induced by the addition of a small deadspace to the ventilator circuit (Levene *et al.*, 1988). The results showed a median rise in anterior cerebral artery velocity of 44% per kPa carbon dioxide tension. This increased to 53% on the second day of life and was reduced by indomethacin therapy. That the response to carbon dioxide is exaggerated in infants when compared to adults was supported by work using radioactive Xenon in preterm infants (67% per kPa, Greisen & Trojaborg, 1987), although some ventilated preterm infants showed a reduced response of 11% per kPa (Pryds *et al.*, 1989) The same group described a 30% per kPa change some years later (Pryds *et al.*, 1990a). Much of the change is due to alteration in blood pressure consequent on variation in carbon dioxide tension (Fenton *et al.*, 1992), and the same confounding problem has been noted in newborn piglets (Rennie *et al.*, 1990; Haaland *et al.*, 1995) and in preterm humans (Menke *et al.*, 1993). No significant differences in reactivity could be demonstrated between healthy and pathological states, although vasoparalysis during carbon dioxide changes has been demonstrated with radioactive xenon in preterm infants with periventricular haemorrhage and term infants with birth asphyxia (Pryds *et al.*, 1989; Pryds *et al.*, 1990b).

Oxygen

Transient hyperoxia was accompanied by a small fall in CBFV (of the order of 1% per kPa rise in oxygen) in both preterm and term infants (Niijima *et al.*, 1988). In term infants hyperoxia caused a change in ventilation and hence in carbon dioxide tension which accounted for almost all the reactivity. Term infants restored their CBFV to normal immediately after the experiment, which was not the case for the preterm babies. Hypoxic hypoxia reduced CBFV in the neonatal lambs studied by Rosenberg *et al.* (1985) but absolute values of CBF could not be predicted from velocity and PI was equally unhelpful. The effect of oxgen on CBFV was ten times smaller than that of carbon dioxide (Menke *et al.*, 1993).

Viscosity of blood

Changes in CBF and CBFV have been demonstrated after both transfusion and haemodilution and are presumed to be due to a change in viscosity (Rosenkrantz *et al.*, 1984; Muizelaar *et al.*, 1986; Ramaekers *et al.*, 1992; Mandelbaum *et al.*, 1994). In cats destruction of the caudate nucleus in polycythaemia reduced CBF values that were restored by dilution and this was thought to represent loss of 'viscosity autoregulation' (Maertzdorf *et al.*, 1989). Blood transfusion can possibly shift the autoregulatory zone upwards, as assessed by CBFV response to blood pressure rises measured with oscillometry during feeding in five infants (Ramaekers *et al.*, 1992).

Blood pressure: autoregulation

The effect of an increase in blood pressure has not been studied directly because of ethical constraints, but there was no change in mean CBFV

Table 5.2. *Validation studies using Doppler ultrasound*

Reference	Species	N	Cerebral blood flow method	Doppler method	Artery	Comment
Guldvog et al. (1980)	adult golden retrievers	3	electromagnetic flowmeter	UNIDOP	common carotid	Good correlation
Busija et al. (1981)	adult cats and dogs	12 7	microspheres	implanted pulsed wave	pial artery	excellent results but measured diameter using a microscope
Batton et al. (1983)	neonatal dogs	30	C14 autoradiography	Parks CW 5 MHz	? ACA	good correlation, esp systolic velocity PI no good.
Hansen et al. (1983)	piglets	9	microspheres	Sonicaid CW 8 MHz pencil	ACA	good, but area under the curve-pooled results
Lundell et al. (1984)	pulsatile flow rig	n/a	absolute values	Vingmed CW range gated	n/a	very good correlations
Greisen et al. (1984)	human neonates	16	xenon 133	CW and range gated pulsed wave	ACA	best with range gated, quite good correlations.
Rosenberg et al. (1985)	newborn lambs	11	microspheres	Medasonics CW 8 MHz	ACA	best correlation with end diastolic flow. PI weak.
Bishop et al. (1986)	human patients	17	xenon 133	EME 2 MHz pulsed	MCA	poor correlation velocity + CBF but very good percentage change with CO_2

Study	Model	n	Comparison method	Doppler device	Artery	Findings
Miles et al. (1987)	pulsatile flow rig	n/a	flowmeter	Medasonics 5 Mhz CW	n/a	good correlations AUTC, PI, PuI, mean
Sonesson & Herin (1988)	newborn lambs	8	radioactive microscope	CW range-gated Vingmed	internal carotid	good correlation CO_2 changes. Doppler predicted 55% change
Morris et al. (1989)	adult cats	6	hydrogen clearance	CW 9 MHz with spectral analysis	MCA	poor correlations – changes achieved by introduction of CO_2 gas
Martin et al. (1990)	newborn lambs – awake	14	radioactive microsphere	ATL Mk 600 duplex	ACA	blood pressure changes – dopamine, etc. fair correlation wide CIs
Rennie et al. (1990)	neonatal piglets	6	hydrogen clearance	CW 9 MHz with spectral anlaysis	MCA	fair correlation when change induced by blood pressure not CO_2
Spencer et al. (1991)	pulsatile rig	n/a	absolute values	8 MHz CW Vasoflo-3	n/a	linear relation with velocity until v low values. PI no good
Haaland et al. (1994)	piglets	9	electromagnetic flowmeter	Vingmed 10 MHz pulsed	internal carotid	good correlations with CO_2 and blood pressure changes
Thoresen et al. (1994)	piglets	5	electromagnetic flowmeter	Vingmed 10 MHz pulsed	internal carotid	fair correlations except during extremes

CW: continuous wave; ATL: Advanced Technology Laboratories; ACA anterior cerebral arteries; MCA: middle cerebral arteries; PI: Pourcelot index; CBF: cerebral blood flow; AUTC: area under the curve; PuI: pulsatility index; CI: confidence interval.

following commencement of dopamine in a small group of preterm infants in whom this form of cardiovascular support reduced the variability of CBFV (Rennie, 1989). Seizures caused an increase in systemic blood pressure, intracranial pressure and CBFV (Perlman & Volpe, 1983). Serial Doppler studies on 32 infants were classified as showing autoregulation if the CBFV remained stable through changes in mean arterial blood pressure of 5 mm Hg or greater (Ahmann *et al.*, 1983). There was no difference in the incidence of periventricular haemorrhage between the groups classified in this way. Jorch & Jorch (1987) studied 23 neonates who collapsed, both during the deterioration and the subsequent course. The mean percentage change in CBFV was 3.3% for each mmHg change in blood pressure for those below 30 weeks gestation and 1% for those above, suggesting impaired autoregulation in these sick, very preterm babies. The same group found a 7.5% per kPa change in a further group of 16 ventilated preterm infants, but there was variability and some interdependence with carbon dioxide changes (Menke *et al.*, 1993). In a study of 48 healthy Dutch infants of less than 32 weeks gestation CBFV was stable in the narrow blood pressure range 31–40 mmHg (Van de Bor & Walther 1991b). Tilting produced a uniphasic response in CBFV in some infants and a biphasic response in others, possibly reflecting presence and absence of autoregulation (Anthony *et al.*, 1993). The type of response was not helpful in predicting later cerebral injury, and several infants showed both types of response at different times. Computerised coherent averaging was used to superimpose CBFV responses to small spontaneous transient increases in blood pressure occuring over a four-minute period, and two clearly different responses emerged (Panerai *et al.*, 1995). In one group of infants the CBFV returned to baseline within 2 seconds,whereas in another the resultant rise persisted. The pattern of a rapid return to baseline was more frequently seen in mature infants. The important question of whether or not autoregulation is present and functioning rapidly in sick infants remains open.

Patent ductus arteriosus

The original observation that patent ductus arteriosus (PDA) could be associated with a reverse flow in the anterior cerebral arteries (Fig. 5.6) was made in 1981 (Perlman *et al.*, 1981). Since then this observation has been confirmed many times and reverse flow has also been seen in the descending aorta (Lipman *et al.*, 1982; Martin *et al.*, 1982; Wilcox *et al.*, 1983). The normal closure of the ductus in term infants was accompanied by a fall in PI but reverse flow was not seen (Wright *et al.*, 1988). Batton *et al.* (1992) felt that closure of a physiologic ductus at term did not influence CBFV. Change in CBFV associated with PDA may provide a sensitive index with which to follow the size of the shunt (van Bel *et al.*, 1987a). In a prospective study of 120 preterm infants in Leicester, 70% had echocardiographic evidence of ductal patency sometime during the first week, mainly on the first day of life. Nineteen (27%) of the infants with

PDA had retrograde flow, on at least one occasion, and there were more infants with retrograde flow in the group who developed periventricular leukomalacia (Shortland *et al.*, 1990a). The evidence for an association between PDA and brain damage was first suggested by Bejar *et al.* (1982) but there was no difference in the outcome for a group of extremely low birthweight infants who underwent prophylactic ductal ligation soon after birth (Cassady *et al.*, 1989). Surgical ligation of the ductus in preterm neonates caused a 50% increase in mean CBFV associated with a change in diastolic velocity and blood pressure (Sonesson *et al.*, 1986). A truly reverberating CBFV may be due to brain death (McMenamin & Volpe, 1983; Hassler *et al.*, 1988) but should be interpreted with caution if the infant has any evidence of PDA.

Variability of cerebral blood flow velocity

From the early days it was apparent that there was often a considerable degree of beat-to-beat variability in CBFV recordings. Perlman *et al.* (1983) recognised that the variability sometimes mirrored that seen in blood pressure, and suggested that high variability might be a factor in the genesis of periventricular haemorrhage. With the availability of recordings made over a period of one minute or more it has become apparent that the variation in CBFV is occuring at several cyclical frequencies (Myers *et al.*, 1987; Anthony *et al.*, 1991; Coughtrey *et al.*, 1992). Figures 5.7(a–c) shows the evolution of the patterns of variability in a short recording and in longer recordings (where the mean velocity of each beat is shown rather than the whole sonogram) lasting one and four minutes. The presence of variation is perhaps not surprising as variations are known to occur in most physiological parameters such as heart rate, respiration and blood pressure. Cyclical variations have also been observed in the CBFV of animals and adult humans, both healthy and head-injured (Mautner *et al.*, 1989, Newell *et al.*, 1992). Attempts to quantify the degree of variability have included the coefficient of the area under the curve of the Doppler sonogram (Perlman *et al.*, 1983; Rennie *et al.*, 1987); the coefficient of variation of the calculated velocity of each cardiac cycle (Cowan & Thoresen, 1987) and the interquartile range of the peak systolic and end-diastolic velocity (Mullaart *et al.*, 1992). Most of the early studies used only 20 cardiac cycles, but longer recordings can be subjected to fast Fourier transformation (FFT). This method has shown that the components of variability include respiration-associated variation (Bignall *et al.*, 1988) as well as the lower frequency variations (corresponding to Lundberg B waves) which result from autonomic nervous system control of vascular tone and thermoregulation. Pial windows in cats reveal that small cerebral arteries are oscillating in size at a similar frequency (Auer & Sayama, 1983). A marked respiratory influence in CBFV shown using FFT spectral analysis was more likely in infants of lower gestation who were artificially ventilated and perhaps resulted from entrainment of naturally occuring varia-

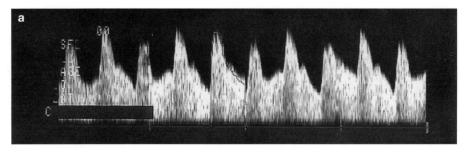

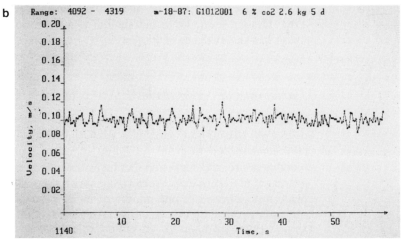

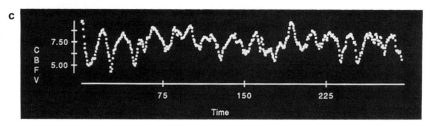

Fig. 5.7. *Illustration of variability in cerebral blood flow velocity recordings: (a) the tracing is only eight seconds long; the whole Doppler spectrum is shown. In the two longer recordings of one (b) and four (c) minutes the mean velocity is plotted for each cardiac cycle.*

bility (Coughtrey *et al.*, 1993). A marked respiratory influence may also reflect hypovolaemia (Rennie, 1989). There was a shift of the power of the FFT spectrum from the low frequency range to that of the respirator frequency when infants were artificially ventilated, also suggesting entrainment (Zernikow *et al.*, 1994). The existence of the entrainment phenomenon suggests that the control systems are non-linear. Oscillations in CBFV do not always occur exactly in phase with those of blood pressure and intracranial pressure, and further study of these relationships may shed light on the normal and abnormal control systems.

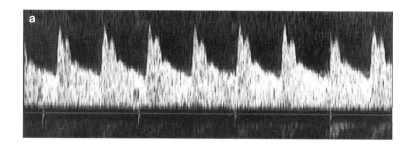

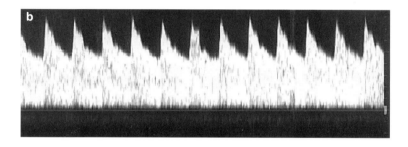

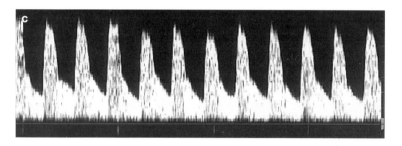

Fig. 5.8. *Examples of cerebral blood flow velocity from a normal infant (a), an infant with birth asphyxia (b) and an infant with hydrocephalus (c) showing the difference in velocity and Pourcelot index.*

Doppler studies in newborn brain injury

Birth asphyxia

Hassler *et al.* (1988) have described in detail the consecutive changes occuring with progressively raised intracranial pressure after cerebral injury, ending with reversed diastolic flow velocity at brain death. Reversed diastolic flow is seen in extremes of brain injury in the newborn but interpretation needs to be cautious as the pattern has also been seen in association with a large left to right shunt through a patent ductus ateriosus. In birth asphyxia the characteristic pattern, usually seen on the second day, is that of raised diastolic velocity. Figure 5.8(a) shows a normal CBFV pattern and Fig. 5.8(b) is an example of a trace from an asphyxiated

89

baby. The velocity is higher, and the diastolic component is markedly increased. A PI below 0.55 has been shown to predict adverse outcome after birth asphyxia (Archer *et al.*, 1986b), and this has been confirmed in three further cases (Yoshida-Shuto *et al.*, 1992). A high velocity also predicts poor outcome (Levene *et al.*, 1989). The abnormal result was obtained after 24 hours, and could represent luxury perfusion. Van Bel *et al.*, (1987b) also found a high velocity and reduced PI in a group of 17 infants, between 32 and 48 hours of life, which was significantly different from controls with hypoxic–ischaemic encephalopathy.

Preterm brain injury

Apart from the work in birth asphyxia, and one study which suggested a relationship between reversed diastolic flow and subsequent ischaemic injury in preterms (Shortland *et al.*, 1990a), CBFV has not proved a very useful predictor of brain injury in the short- or long-term (Shortland *et al.*, 1990b). This is true even when more complex analysis such as carbon dioxide reactivity has been studied (Fenton *et al.*, 1992). Prediction of long-term outcome has also been tried: a high PI correlated with an adverse outcome in a group of 60 preterm infants followed in Leiden (Van Bel *et al.*, 1989a). Recently in Cambridge, UK, we followed a cohort of very low birthweight infants to 18 months. Nine were significantly handicapped. The CBFV failed to predict any adverse outcome when compared to the more easily obtained cranial ultrasound image (Rennie *et al.*, 1995).

Brain death

The requirements for the diagnosis of brain death are extraordinarily difficult to fulfil in the newborn (Volpe, 1987). Absent CBF is obviously associated with loss of cerebral function but few users of Doppler ultrasound would be sufficiently confident to pronounce that there was undoubtedly no CBF when the consequence could be withdrawal of artificial ventilation. Ashwal & Schneider (1989) have suggested that the American Task Force guidelines (Task Force, 1987) including neurological assessment, electrical silence and isotope demonstration of absent CBF can be applied to the preterm and term newborn but also point out that true brain death is rare in this group. McMenamin & Volpe (1983), Ahmann *et al.* (1987) Kirkham *et al.* (1987) and Bode *et al.* (1988) have described the Doppler appearances in brain death in infants , and these have evolved into a description of a characteristic and easily recognisable 'reverberating' flow pattern. There is short-lasting and low velocity forward flow counterbalanced by substantial retrograde flow in early diastole. This may be followed by a further period of forward flow in late diastole, although this is not always described and may be the most important distinguishing feature (Hayashi *et al.*, 1992a).

Hydrocephalus

Although all studies report an increase in the PI in post-haemorrhagic hydrocephalus and in other forms of congenital hydrocephalus (Chadduck *et al.*, 1989) the correlation between the PI and intracranial pressure does not seem reliable enough for Doppler to be used as a predictive clinical tool. The relationship with velocity has been poor, perhaps due to distortion of the vessels (Finn *et al.*, 1990). Different authors have found different reasons for the increase in PI, some with a reduction of end-diastolic and some finding a raised systolic velocity. There is usually a wide overlap between the normal and abnormal groups, and this led Quinn *et al.* (1992) to state that they were unable to define an action line. Most of the studies report opportunistic observations immediately before and after shunting, rather than studying the evolution of hydrocephalus. There is thus little information on the earliest postnatal age at which a Doppler study might be useful, although the change in PI occurs early. Doppler studies may give more information than measurement of sequential changes in ventricular size from ultrasound scan images (Levene & Starte, 1981) or plotting the head circumference on a chart, but this has yet to be convincingly demonstrated. The methodology used has varied considerably, as can be seen in Table 5.3, which gives a summary of the literature. Figure 5.8(a–c) shows examples of the difference in CBFV between normal infants (a) and those with asphyxia (b) and hydrocephalus (c).

Drug studies

Surfactant

Several studies have shown changes in CBFV after instillation of surfactant, albeit in different directions. Van de Bor *et al.* (1991) studied the administration of the synthetic surfactant Exosurf as rescue treatment in 25 preterm babies. Mean flow velocity increased by 33% at 5 minutes, returning to baseline values by 30 minutes. The change was associated with a small increase in blood pressure and arterial oxygen tension. Cowan *et al.* (1991) showed an immediate 33% fall in CBFV and blood pressure following the administration of the natural porcine surfactant Curosurf as rescue therapy. The change lasted for about 20 minutes and was most marked in the diastolic velocity, leading the authors to speculate that there was increased shunting through the ductus leading to cerebral steal. Halliday *et al.* (1989) could not demonstrate an increase in pulmonary blood flow after the administration of porcine surfactant although this has subsequently been thought to occur, using Doppler to demonstrate tricuspid regurgitation (Kaapa *et al.*, 1992, 1993). In Leiden, when Curosurf was given to 14 babies as prophylaxis after birth (Van Bel *et al.*, 1992) there was a slight fall in blood pressure and mean CBFV in the internal carotid

Table 5.3. *Doppler ultrasound studies in neonatal hydrocephalus*

Reference	No. of subjects	Doppler instrument	Artery	Result
Hill & Volpe (1982)	11	Medasonics CW zero cross	ACA	PI raised (0.9) decreased end diastolic
Alvisi et al. (1985)	10	Angiodop 481 CW system	ACA	raised PI (0.76), increased systolic velocity
Van Bel et al. (1988 b)	10	Parks CW zero crossing	ACA	Reduction in PI (0.63) after drainage; increased peak velocity
Deeg et al. (1988)	52	duplex pulsed	ACA	9 without progression HC normal: 17 progressive increase in PI due to reduced diastolic
Fischer & Livingstone (1989)	9	2 MHz Acuson 128 duplex	MCA	RI increased, reduced after VPS; RI varied with pressure; absent end–diastolic flow
Chadduck et al. (1989)	46	Acuson 128 Dupex colour	MCA, ACA	PI increased before shunts (0.84 vs 0.74 HC no VPS)
Seibert et al. (1989)	8	Acuson 128 duplex colour	MCA, ACA	PI increased (0.9), correlation with ICP in dogs
Lui et al. (1990b)	9	ATL Mk 450 range gated	ACA	increase in PI; absent or reversed end–diastolic velocity in 6: 4–6 required shunts

Nishimaki et al. (1990)	11	Yokogawa duplex system	ACA, basilar	PI increased (0.84); ratio ACA/basilar >1.0
Pople et al. (1991)	63	EME TC 64	MCA	PI correlated with ICP and 56% of children with blocked shunt had raised PI versus 3% not blocked
Goh et al. (1991)	14	Doptek PW	MCA	RI decreased after taps poor correlation with ICP; not all neonates
Quinn et al. (1992)	18	Acuson 128 Duplex colour	ACA + veins	PI increased (0.8), NSD in velocity, no correlation ICP
Quinn & Pople (1992)	62	EME TC 64	MCA	same results, same patients as Pople et al. (1991)
Goh et al. (1992a)	18	Diasonics duplex	ACA, MCA	PI increased (0.9), correlation ICP for MCA only
Goh et al. (1992b)	7	Doptek pulsed wave	MCA	sleep studies – some raised CBV with raised ICP some reduced.
Kempley & Gamsu (1993b)	6	duplex HP	ACA & MCA	reduced PI increased velocity after taps

ATL: Advanced Technology Laboratories; ACA: anterior cerebral artery; VPS: ventriculoperitoneal shunt; CW: continuous wave; MCA: middle cerebral artery; RI: resistance index; PI: Pourcelot index; ICP: intracranial pressure; NSD: no significant difference; HC: hydrocephalus; CBV: cerebral blood velocity.

Table 5.4. *Summary of the studies on the effects of indomethacin on cerebral blood flow velocity in the newborn*

Reference	No. of subjects	Equipment	Artery	Result
Cowan 1986	3	6 MHz CW	ACA	50% reduction in velocity
Evans *et al.* (1987)	5	ATL, Mk 600 duplex range-gated	ACA	BP increased 15% CBF reduced 60% by 1 min still 35% below by 60 min
Laudignon *et al.* (1988)	13	Medasonics CW	ACA	22% fall by 15 min sustained by 120 min – effect first dose only
Pryds *et al.* (1988)	6	Xenon 133	total CBF	rapid fall in global CBF 22%
Lundell *et al.* (1989)	7 (lambs) 10 infants	Vingmed 5MHz duplex	internal carotid	25–40% reduction after 60 minutes
Van Bel *et al.* (1989b)	24	Parks CW 9.6 or or 5 MHz zero–crossing	ACA	immediate fall lasting 2 hours; normal by 3 hours
Colditz *et al.* (1989a)	12	Angioscan III	ACA	CBFV reduced: only during rapid infusion.
Edwards *et al.* (1990)	13 (some slowly)	NIRS	–	CBF, CB volume fell in both groups by 30 min.
Mardoum *et al.* (1991)	7 (and 8 controls)	ATL range-gated	internal carotid	Fall in CBFV immediately, lasting 90 min + fall in BP.
Austin *et al.* (1992)	11	Hewlett Packard range-gated, 5 MHz	ACA and MCA	slow infusion slow reduction; larger change in MCA

ACA: anterior cerebral arteries; MCA: middle cerebral arteries; BP: blood pressure; CBF: cerebral blood flow; CBFV: cerebral blood flow velocity; CB: cerebral blood.

artery associated with an increase in fluctuation of the velocity pattern. After 10 minutes the velocity rose above baseline. A fall in blood pressure and a supression of electrical activity in the brain has also been noted after surfactant administration (Hellstrom–Westas *et al.*, 1992). Jorch *et al.* (1989) failed to find any change in CBFV when measured 10 minutes before and after prophylactic surfactant administration, although he also noticed an increase in variability. A stable CBFV, blood pressure and cardiac output at 20 minutes after very slow administration of surfactant (Exosurf 50 mg = 5 ml.kg^{-1}) was recorded by Saliba *et al* (1992). Rey *et al.* (1994) claimed that 100 mg.kg^{-1} of Curosurf produced no change in blood pressure or CBFV whereas 200 mg.kg^{-1} was followed by a fall in both. The fact that any change in cerebral blood volume after surfactant therapy is insignificant was stressed by Edwards *et al.* (1992) using near infra-red spectroscopy.

Indomethacin

In all the published studies, indomethacin has been shown to reduce CBFV in human newborns. Some claim that the effect is less if the drug is given slowly. The change lasts for at least an hour, and seems to be an effect of the drug rather than the change in the circulation achieved by closure of the ductus, as surgical closure produces a change in the opposite direction (Sonesson *et al.*, 1986; Saliba *et al.*, 1991). Surgical closure also increases the blood pressure, which tends to be reduced in infants with PDA. Table 5.4 summarises the results and includes some studies which used other methods such as near infra red spectroscopy (Edwards *et al.*, 1990).

Acetazolamide

Acetazolamide is known to increase CBF in adults and is given to infants with hydrocephalus. An 86% increase in CBFV measured in the MCA has been reported to occur in infants (Cowan & Whitelaw, 1991). The change was only reported after the first intravenous dose which was also associated with a rise in arterial carbon dioxide tension.

Caffeine and aminophylline

Aminophylline causes a reduction of CBFV in adults, and a 25% reduction was recorded after an intravenous dose given to infants by Rosenkrantz & Oh (1984) and Chang & Gray (1994). Chang & Gray (1994) also pointed out that aminophylline therapy reduces carbon dioxide levels. Near infra-red spectroscopy confirmed the Doppler results (McDonnell *et al.*, 1992). Aminophylline at therapeutic serum concentrations was not associated with a reduction in CBFV in the sudy by Ghai *et al.* (1989), and the change in CBF measured with radioactive xenon was apparently too small to affect cerebral function (Pryds & Schneider, 1991). Caffeine therapy caused a reduction in carbon dioxide tensions 24 hours after administration but no change in CBFV (Van Bel *et al.*, 1989c).

Analgesia and sedation

Phenobarbitone reduced CBF measured with radioactive microspheres in a group of ketamine anaesthetised newborn puppies (Goddard–Finegold *et al.*, 1990), but has not been associated with any significant alteration of haemodynamics in human newborns (Saliba *et al.*, 1992), nor could this drug be shown to reduce fluctuating CBFV (Kuban *et al.*, 1988). Thiopentone has been shown to reduce CBFV in older children with head injuries (De Bray *et al.*, 1993). Diazepam also appears to be safe in this respect (Jorch *et al.*, 1990b). Variability of CBFV was reduced by morphine and pancuronium paralysis in one small study (Colditz *et al.*, 1989b). A small fall in blood pressure and CBFV was noted after midazolam (Van Straaten *et al.*, 1992).

References

Aaslid, R., Markwalder, T-M. & Nornes, H. (1982) Noninvasive transcranial Doppler ultrasound recording of flow velocity in the basal cerebral arteries. *Journal of Neurosurgery*, **57**:769–74.

Ahmann, P.A., Dykes, F.D., Lazzara, A., Holt, P.J., Giddens, D.P. & Carrigan, T.A. (1983) Relationship between pressure passivity and subependymal/intraventricular hemorrhage as assessed by pulsed Doppler ultrasound. *Pediatrics*, **72**:665–9.

Ahmann, P.A., Carrigan, T.A., Carlton, D., Wyly, B. & Schwartz, J.F. (1987) Brain death in children: characteristic common carotid arterial velocity patterns measured with pulsed Doppler ultrasound. *Journal of Pediatrics*, **110**:723–8.

Alvisi, C., Cerisoli, M., Giulioni, M., Monari, P., Salvioli, G.P., Sandri, F., Lippi, C., Bovicelli, L. & Pilu, G. (1985) Evaluation of cerebral blood flow changes by transfontanelle Doppler ultrasound in infantile hydrocephalus. *Child's Nervous System*, **1**:244–7.

Ando, Y., Takashima, S. & Takeshita, K. (1983) Postnatal changes in cerebral blood flow velocity in normal term neonates. *Brain Development*, **5**:525–8.

Ando, Y., Takashima, S. & Takeshita, K. (1985) Cerebral blood flow velocity in preterm neonates. *Brain Development*, **7**:385–91.

Anthony, M.Y., Evans, D.H. & Levene, M.I. (1991) Cyclical variations in cerebral blood flow velocity. *Archives of Disease in Childhood*, **66**:12–16.

Anthony, M.Y., Evans, D.H. & Levene, M.I. (1993) Neonatal cerebral blood flow velocity responses to changes in posture. *Archives of Disease in Childhood*, **69**:304–8.

Archer, L.N.J., Evans, D.H. & Levene, M.I. (1985) Doppler ultrasound examination of the anterior cerebral arteries of normal newborn infants – the effect of postnatal age. *Early Human Development* **10**:255–60.

Archer, L.N.J., Evans, D.H., Paton, J.Y. & Levene, M.I. (1986a) Controlled hypercapnia and neonatal cerebral artery Doppler ultrasound waveforms. *Pediatric Research*, **20**:218–21.

Archer, L.N.J., Levene, M.I. & Evans, D.H. (1986b) Cerebral artery Doppler ultrasonography for prediction of outcome after perinatal asphyxia. *Lancet*, ii: 1116–18.

Ashwal, S. & Schneider, S. (1989) Brain death in the newborn. *Pediatrics*, 84:429–437.

Auer, L.M. & Sayama, I. (1983) Intracranial pressure oscillations (B waves) caused by oscillations in cerebrovascular volume. *Acta Neurochir*, 68:93–100.

Austin, N.C., Pairaudeau, P.W., Hames, T.K. & Hall, M.A. (1992) Regional cerebral blood flow velocity changes after indomethacin infusion in preterm infants. *Archives of Disease in Childhood*, 67:851–4.

Bada, H.S., Hajjar, W., Chua, C. & Sumner, D.S. (1979) Non invasive diagnosis of neonatal asphyxia and intraventricular haemorrhage using Doppler ultrasound. *Journal of Pediatrics*, 95:775–9.

Batton, D.G., Hellman, J. & Hernandez, M.D. (1983) Regional cerebral blood flow, cerebral blood flow velocity and pulsatility index in newborn dogs. *Pediatric Research*, 17:908–12.

Batton, D.G., Riordan, S. & Riggs, T. (1992) Cerebral blood flow velocity in normal, full term newborns is not related to ductal closure. *American Journal of Diseases in Children*, 146:737–40.

Bejar, R., Merritt, T.A. & Coen, R.W. (1982) Pulsatility index, patent ductus arteriosus and brain damage. *Pediatrics*, 69:818–22.

Bignall, S., Bailey, P.C., Rivers, R.P.A. & Lissauer, T.J. (1988) Quantification of cardiovascular instability in premature infants using spectral analysis of waveforms. *Pediatric Research*, 23:398–401.

Bishop, C.C.R., Powell, S., Rutt, D. & Browse, N.L. (1986) Transcranial Doppler measurement of middle cerebral artery blood flow velocity: a validation study. *Stroke*, 17:913–15.

Bode, H. & Wais, U. (1988) Age dependence of flow velocities in basal cerebral arteries. *Archives of Disease in Childhood*, 62:606–11.

Bode, H,. Sauer, M. & Pringsheim, W. (1988) Diagnosis of brain stem death by transcranial Doppler sonography. *Archives of Disease in Childhood*, 63:1474–8.

Busija, D.W., Heistad, D.D. & Marcus, M.L. (1981) Continuous measurements of cerebral blood flow in anesthetized cats and dogs. *American Journal of Physiology*, 241:H228–H234.

Calvert, S.A., Ohlsson, A., Hosking, M.C., Erskine, L., Fong, K. & Shennan, A.T. (1988) Serial measurements of cerebral blood flow velocity in preterm infants during the first 72 hours of life. *Acta Paediatrica Scandinavica*, 77:625–31.

Cassady, G., Grouse, D.T., Kirklin, J.W., Strange, M.J., Joiner, C.H., Godoy, G., Odrezin, G.T., Cutter, G.R., Kirklin, J.K., Pacifico, A., Collins, M.V., Lell, W.A., Satterwhite, C. & Philips, J.B. (1989) Randomised controlled trial of very early prophylactic ligation of the ductus arteriosus in babies who weighed 1000 g or less at birth. *New England Journal of Medicine*, 320:1511–16.

Chadduck, W.M. Seibert, J.J., Adametz, J., Glasier, C.M., Crabtree, M. & Stansell, C.A. (1989) Cranial Doppler ultrasonography correlates with criteria for ventriculoperitoneal shunting. *Surgical Neurology* 31:122–8.

Chang, J. & Gray, P.H. (1994) Aminophylline therapy and cerebral blood flow velocity in preterm infants. *Journal of Pediatrics and Child Health*, 30:123–5.

Cheung, Y.F., Lam, P.K.L. & Yeung, C.Y. (1994) Early postnatal cerebral Doppler changes in relation to birthweight. *Early Human Development*, 37:57–66.

Colditz, P., Murphy, D., Rolfe, P. & Wilkinson, A.R. (1989a) Effect of infusion rate of indomethacin on cerebrovascular responses in preterm infants. *Archives of Disease in Childhood*, **64**:8–12.

Colditz, P., Williams, G.L., Berry, A.B. & Symonds, P.J. (1989b) Variability of Doppler flow velocity and cerebral perfusion pressure is reduced in the neonate by sedation and neuromuscular blockade. *Australian Journal of Pediatrics*, **25**:171–3.

Connors, G., Hunse, C., Gagon, R., Richardson, B., Han, V. & Rosenberg, H. (1992) Perinatal assessment of cerebral blood flow velocity wave forms in the human fetus and neonate. *Pediatric Research*, **31**:649–52.

Coughtrey, H., Rennie, J.M. & Evans, D. H. (1992) Postnatal evolution of slow variations in cerebral blood flow velocity. *Archives of Disease in Childhood*, **67**:412–15.

Coughtrey, H., Rennie, J.M., Evans, D. H. & Cole, T.J., (1993) Factors associated with respiration induced variability in cerebral blood flow velocity. *Archives of Disease in Childhood*, **68**: 312–16.

Cowan, F., (1986) Indomethacin, patent ductus and cerebral blood flow velocities. *Journal of Pediatrics*, **109**: 341–4.

Cowan, F. & Thoresen, M. (1987) The effects of intermittent positive pressure ventilation on cerebral arterial and venous blood velocities in the newborn infant. *Acta Paediatrica Scandinavica*, **76**:239–47.

Cowan, F. & Whitelaw, A. (1991) Acute effects of acetazolamide on cerebral blood velocity and $PaCO_2$ in newborn infants. *Acta Paediatrica Scandinavica*, **80**:22–7.

Cowan, F., Whitelaw, A., Wertheim, D. & Silverman, M. (1991) Cerebral blood flow velocity changes after rapid administration of surfactant. *Archives of Disease in Childhood*, **66**: 1105–09.

De Bray, J.M., Granry, J.C., Monrigal, J.P., Leftheriotis, G. & Saumet, J.L. (1993) Effects of thiopental on middle cerebral artery blood velocities: a transcranial Doppler study in children. *Child's Nervous System*, **9**:220–3.

Deeg, K.H., Paul, T., Rupprecht, Th., Harms, D. & Mang, C. (1988) Gepulste dopplersonographische Bestimmung absoluter gflubgeschwingkeiten in der ateria cerebri anterior bein Sauglingen mit Hydrocephalus im Vergleich zu einem gesundedn Kontrollkollektiv. *Monatsschrift für Kinderheilkunde*, **136**: 85–94.

Deeg, K.H. & Rupprecht, Th. (1989) Pulsed Doppler sonographic measurements of normal values for the flow velocities in the intracranial arteries of healthy newborns. *Pediatric Radiology*, **19**:71–7.

Drayton, M.R. & Skidmore, R. (1987) Vasoactivity of the major intracranial arteries in newborn infants. *Archives of Disease in Childhood*, **62**:236–40.

Edwards, A.D., Wyatt, J.S., Richardson, C., Potter, A., Cope, M., Delphy, D.T. & Reynolds, E.O.R. (1990) Effects of indomethacin on cerebral haemodynamics in very preterm infants. *Lancet*, **335**: 1491–5.

Edwards, A.D., McCormick, D.C., Roth, S.C., Elwell, C.E., Peebles, D.M., Cope, M., Wyatt, J.S., Delphy, D.T. & Reynolds, E.O.R. (1992) Cerebral haemodynamic effects of treatment with modified natural surfactant investigated by near infra-red spectroscopy. *Pediatric Research*, **32**:532–6.

Evans, D.H. (1985) On measurement of mean velocity of flow using Doppler ultrasound. *Ultrasound in Medicine and Biology*, **11**:735–41.

Evans, D.H., Levene, M.I. & Archer, L.N.J., (1987) The effect of indomethacin on cerebral blood flow velocity in premature infants. *Developmental Medicine and Child Neurology*, **29**: 776–82

Evans, D.H., Levene, M.I., Shortland, D.B. & Archer, L.N.J. (1988) Resistance index, blood flow velocity and resistance area product in the cerebral arteries of very low birthweight infants during the first week of life. *Ultrasound in Medicine and Biology*, **14**:103–10.

Fenton, A.C., Shortland, D.B., Papathoma, E., Evans, D.H. & Levene, M.I. (1990) Normal range for blood flow velocity in cerebral arteries of newly born term infants. *Early Human Development*, **22**:73–9.

Fenton, A.C., Papathoma, E., Evans, D.H. & Levene, M.I. (1991) Neonatal cerebral venous flow velocity measurement using a colour flow Doppler system. *Journal of Clinical Ultrasound*, **19**:69–72.

Fenton, A.C., Woods, K.L., Evans, D.H. & Levene, M.I. (1992) Cerebrovascular carbon dioxide reactivity and failure of autoregulation in preterm infants. *Archives of Disease in Childhood*, **67**:835–9.

Ferrari, F., Kelsall, A.W.R., Rennie, J.M. & Evans, D.H. (1994) The relationship between cerebral blood flow velocity and sleep state in normal newborns. *Pediatric Research*, **35**:50–4.

Finn, J.P., Quinn, M.W., Hall-Craggs, M.A. & Kendall, B.E. (1990) Impact of vessel distortion on transcranial Doppler velocity measurements correlation with magnetic resonance imaging. *Journal of Neurosurgery*, **73**:572–5

Fischer, A.Q. & Livingstone, J.N. (1989) Transcranial Doppler and real-time cranial sonography in neonatal hydrocephalus. *Journal of Child Neurology*, **4**:64–9

Fischer, A.Q., Taormina, M.A., Akhtar, B. & Chandley, B.A. (1991) The effect of sleep on intracranial haemodynamics: a transcranial Doppler study. *Journal of Child Neurology* **6**:155–8.

Ghai, V., Raju, T.N.K., Kim, S.Y. & McCulloch, K.M. (1989) Regional cerebral blood flow velocity after aminophylline therapy in premature newborn infants. *Journal of Pediatrics*, **114**:870–3.

Goddard-Finegold, J., Donley, D., Adham, B.I. & Michael, L.H. (1990) Phenobarbital and cerebral blood flow during hypotension in the newborn beagle. *Pediatrics*, **86**:501–8.

Goh, D., Minns, R.A., Pye, S.D. & Steers, A.J.W. (1991) Cerebral blood flow velocity changes after ventricular taps and ventriculoperitoneal shunts. *Child's Nervous System*, **7**:452–7.

Goh, D., Minns, R.A., Hendry, G.M.A., Thambyayah, M. & Steers, A.J.W. (1992a) Cerebrovascular resistive index assessed by Duplex Doppler sonography and its relationship to intracranial pressure in infantile hydrocephalus. *Pediatric Radiology*, **22**:246–50.

Goh, D., Minns, R.A., Pye, S.D. & Steers, A.J.W. (1992b) Cerebral blood flow velocity and intermittent intracranial pressure elevation during sleep in hydrocephalic children. *Developmental Medicine and Child Neurology*, **34**:676–89.

Gray, P.H., Griffin, E.A., Drumm, J.E., Fitzgerald, D.E. & Duignan, N.M. (1983) Continuous wave Doppler ultrasound in evaluation of cerebral blood flow in neonates. *Archives of Disease in Childhood*, **58**:677–81.

Greisen, G., Johansen, K., Ellison, P.H., Frederiksen, P.S., Mali, J. & Friis-Hansen, B. (1984) Cerebral blood flow in the newborn infant comparison of Doppler ultrasound and Xe-133 clearance. *Journal of Pediatrics*, **104**:411–18.

Greisen, G. & Trojaborg, W. (1987) Cerebral blood flow, $PaCO_2$ changes and visual evoked potentials in mechanically ventilated, preterm infants. *Acta Paediatrica Scandinavica*, **76**:394–400.

Guldvog, I., Kjaernes, M., Thoresen, M. & Walloe, L. (1980) Blood flow in arteries determined transcutaneously by an electronic Doppler velocitymeter as compared to electromagnetic measurements on the exposed vessels. *Acta Physiologica Scandinavica*, **109**:211–16.

Haaland, K., Karlsson, B., Skovlund, E. & Thoresen, M. (1994) Simultaneous measurements of cerebral circulation with electromagnetic flowmetry and Doppler ultrasound velocity in the newborn pig. *Pediatric Research*, **36**:601–6.

Haaland, K., Karlsson, B., Skovlund, E., Lagercrantz, H. & Thoresen, M. (1995) Postnatal development of the cererbral blood flow velocity reponse to changes in CO_2 and MABP in the piglet. *Acta Paediatrica Scandinavica*, **84**:144–20.

Hague, A., Thoresen, M. & Walloe, L. (1980) Changes in cerebral blood flow during hyperventilation and CO_2 breathing measured transcutaneously in humans by a bidirectional pulsed ultrasound Doppler blood velocitymeter. *Acta Physiologica Scandinavica*, **110**:167–73.

Halliday, H., McCord, F.B., McClure, G. & Reid, M. Mc. (1989) Acute effects of instillation of surfactant in severe respiratory distress syndrome. *Archives of Disease in Childhood*, **64**:13–16.

Hansen, N.B., Stonestreet, B.S., Rosenkrantz, T.S. & Oh, W. (1983) Validity of Doppler measurements of anterior cerebral artery blood flow velocity correlation with brain blood flow in piglets. *Pediatrics*, **72**:526–9.

Harper, A.M. & Glass, H.I. (1965) Effect of alterations in the arterial carbon dioxide tension on the blood flow through the cerebral cortex at normal and low arterial blood pressure. *Journal of Neurology, Neurosurgery and Psychiatry*, **28**:449–52.

Hassler, W., Steinmetz, H. & Gawlowski, J. (1988) Transcranial Doppler ultrasonography in raised intracranial pressure and in intracranial circulatory arrest. *Journal of Neurosurgery*, **68**:745–51.

Hayashi, T., Ichiyama, T., Kondoh, O., Tanaka, O., Tateishi, H., Narima, N. & Saitoh, T. (1992a) Reverse flow in the intracranial arteries – the possible significance of comparative flow in the anterior cerebral and the basilar arteries. *Pediatric Radiology*, **22**:128–30.

Hayashi, T., Ichiyama, T., Uchida, M., Tashiro, N. & Tanaka, H. (1992b) Evaluation by colour Doppler and pulsed Doppler sonography of blood flow velocities in intracranial arteries during the early neonatal period. *European Journal of Pediatrics*, **151**:461–5.

Hellstrom-Westas, L., Bell, A.H., Skov, L., Greisen, G. & Svenningsen, N. (1992) Cerebroelectrical depression following surfactant treatment in preterm neonates. *Pediatrics*, **89**:643–7.

Hill, A. & Volpe, J.J. (1982) Decrease in pulsatile flow in the anterior cerebral arteries in infantile hydrocephalus. *Pediatrics*, **69**:4–7.

Jorch, G. & Jorch, N. (1987) Failure of autoregulation of cerebral blood flow in neonates studied by pulsed Doppler ultrasound of the internal carotid artery. *European Journal of Pediatrics*, **146**:468–72.

Jorch, G., Rabe, H., Garbe, M., Michel, E. & Gortner, L. (1989) Acute and protracted effects of intratracheal surfactant application on internal carotid artery blood flow velocity, blood pressure and carbon dioxide tension in very low birthweight infants. *European Journal of Pediatrics*, **148**:770–3.

Jorch, G., Huster, T. & Rabe, H. (1990a) Dependency of Doppler parameters in the anterior cerebral artery on behavioural states in preterm and term neonates. *Biology of the Neonate*, **58**:79–86.

Jorch, G., Rabe, H., Rickers, E., Bomelburg, T. & Hentschel, R. (1990b) Cerebral blood flow velocity assessed by Doppler technique after intravenous application of Diazepam in very low birthweight infants. *Developmental Pharmacology and Therapeutics*, **14**:102–7.

Kaapa, P., Kero, P. & Saraste, M. (1992) Synthetic surfactant replacement therapy decreases estimated pulmonary artery pressure in respiratory distress syndrome. *American Journal of Diseases in Childhood*, **146**:961–4.

Kaapa, P., Seppanen, M., Kero, P. & Saraste, M. (1993) Pulmonary haemodynamics after synthetic surfactant replacement in neonatal respiratory distress syndrome. *Pediatrics*, **123**:115–19.

Kempley, S.T. & Gamsu, H.R. (1993a) Arterial blood pressure and blood flow velocity in major cerebral and visceral arteries. I. Inter-individual differences. *Early Human Development*, **34**:227–32.

Kempley, S.T. & Gamsu, H.R. (1993b) Changes in cerebral blood flow velocity after cerebrospinal fluid drainage. *Archives of Disease in Childhood*, **69**:74–6.

Kirkham, F.J., Padayachee, T.S., Parsons, S., Seargeant, L.S., House, F.R. & Gosling, R.G. (1986) Transcranial measurement of blood velocities in basal cerebral arteries using Doppler ultrasound. *Ultrasound in Medicine and Biology*, **12**:15–21.

Kirkham, F.J., Levin, S.D., Padayachee, T.S., Kyme, M.C., Neville, B.G.R. & Gosling, R.G. (1987) Transcranial pulsed Doppler ultrasound findings in brain stem death. *Journal of Neurology, Neurosurgery and Psychiatry*, **50**;1504–13.

Kuban, K.C.K., Skouteli, H., Cherer, A., Brown, E., Leviton, A., Pagno, M., Allred, E. & Sullivan, K.F. (1988) Hemorrhage, phenobarbital and fluctuating cerebral blood flow velocity in the neonate. *Pediatrics*, **82**:548–53.

Kurmanavichius, J., Rus, W., Mieth, D., Konig, V., Huch, R. & Huch, A. (1991) Effect of postnatal age on blood flow velocity in the middle cerebral artery of very low birthweight infants. *Pediatric Reviews and Communications*, **5**:181–9.

Laudignon, N., Chomtob, S., Bard, H. & Aranda, J.V. (1988) Effect of indomethacin on cerebral blood flow velocity of premature newborns. *Biology of the Neonate*, **54**:254–82.

Levene, M.I. & Starte, D. A. (1981) Longitudinal study of post-haemorrhagic venticular dilatation in the newborn. *Archives of Disease in Childhood*, **56**:905–910.

Levene, M.I., Shortland, D., Gibson, N. & Evans, D.H. (1988) Carbon dioxide reactivity of the cerebral circulation in extremely preterm infants: effects of postnatal age and indomethacin. *Pediatric Research*, **24**:175–9.

Levene, M.I., Fenton, A.C., Evans, D.H., Archer, L.N.J., Shortland, D.B. & Gibson, N.A. (1989) Severe birth asphyxia and abnormal cerebral blood flow velocity. *Developmental Medicine and Child Neurology*, **31**:427–34.

Lipman, A., Serwer, G.A. & Brazy, J.E. (1982) Abnormal cerebral haemodynamics in preterm infants with patent ductus arteriosus. *Pediatrics*, **69**:778–81.

Lui, K., Hellmann, J., Soto, G., Donoghue, V. & Daneman, A. (1990a) Regional cerebral blood flow velocity patterns in newborn infants. *Journal of Pediatrics and Child Health*, **26**:55–7.

Lui, K., Hellmann, J., Sprigg, A. & Daneman, A. (1990b) Cerebral blood flow velocity patterns in post-haemorrhagic ventricular dilatation. *Child's Nervous System*, **6**:250–3.

Lundell, B.W.P., Lindstrom, D.P. & Arnold, T.G. (1984) Neonatal cerebral blood flow velocity I. *Acta Paediatrica Scandinavica*, **73**:810–15.

Lundell, B.W.P., Sonsesson, S-E. & Sundell, H. (1989) Cerebral blood flow following indomethacin administration. *Developmental Pharmacology and Therapeutics*, **13**:139–44.

Maertzdorf, W.J., Tangelder, G.J., Slaaf, D.W. & Blanco, C.E. (1989) Effects of partial plasma exchange transfusion of cerebral blood flow velocity in polycythaemic preterm, term and small for dates newborn infants. *European Journal of Pediatrics*, **148**:774–8.

Mandelbaum, V.H.A., Guajardo, C.D., Nelle, M. & Linderkamp, O. (1994) Effects of polycythaemia and haemodilution on circulation in neonates. *Archives of Disease in Childhood*, **71**:F53–F54.

Mardoum, R., Bejar, R., Merritt, A. & Berry, C. (1991) Controlled study of the effects of indomethacin on cerebral blood flow velocities in newborn infants. *Journal of Pediatrics*, **118**:112–15.

Markwalder, T-M., Grolimund, P., Seiler, R.W., Roth, F. & Aaslid, R. (1984) Dependency of blood flow velocity in the middle cerebral artery on end-tidal carbon dioxide partial pressure – a transcranial ultrasound Doppler study. *Journal of Cerebral Blood Flow and Metabolism* **4**:368–72.

Martin, C.G., Snider, R., Katz, S.M., Peabody, J.L. & Brady, J.P. (1982) Abnormal cerebral blood flow patterns in preterm infants with a large patent ductus arteriosus. *Journal of Pediatrics*, **101**:587–93.

Martin, C.G., Hansen, T.N., Goddard-Finegold, J., LeBlanc, A., Giesler, M.E. & Smith, S. (1990) Prediction of brain blood flow using pulsed Doppler ultrasonography in newborn lambs. *Journal of Clinical Ultrasound*, **18**:487–95.

Mautner, D., Dirnagl, U., Haberl, R., Schmiedek, P., Garner, C., Villringer, A. & Einhaup, K.M. (1989) B waves in healthy persons. In *Intracranial pressure VII*, ed. J.T. Hoff & A.L. Betz, pp. 209–12. Berlin: Springer-Verlag.

McDicken, W.N. (1991) *Diagnostic Ultrasonics*, 3rd edn. Edinburgh: Churchill Livingstone.

McDonnell, M., Ives, N.K. & Hope, P.L. (1992) Intravenous aminophylline and cerebral blood flow in preterm infants. *Archives of Disease in Childhood*, **67**:416–18.

McMenamin, J.B. & Volpe, J.J. (1983) Doppler ultrasonography in the determination of neonatal brain death. *Annals of Neurology*, **14**:302–7.

Meerman, R.J., Van Bel, F., Zwieten, P.H.T., Oepkes, D. & den Ouden, L. (1990) Fetal and neonatal cerebral blood velocity in the normal fetus and neonate a longitudinal Doppler ultrasound study. *Early Human Development*, **24**:209–17.

Menke, J., Michel, E., Rabe, H., Bresser, B.W., Grohs, B., Schnitt, R.M. & Jorch, G. (1993) Simultaneous influence of blood pressure, PCO_2, and PO_2 on cerebral blood flow velocity in preterm infants of less than 33 week's gestation. *Pediatric Research*, **34**:173–7.

Miles, R.D., Menke, J.A., Bashiru, M. & Colliver, J.A. (1987) Relationships of five Doppler measures with flow in an in vitro model and clinical findings in newborn infants. *Journal of Ultrasound in Medicine*, **6**:597–9.

Mires, G.J., Patel, N.B., Forsyth, J.S. & Howie, P.W. (1994) Neonatal cerebral blood flow waveforms in the uncomplicated preterm infant: reference values. *Early Human Development*, **36**:205–12.

Mirro, R. & Gonzalez, M.D. (1987) Perinatal anterior cerebral artery Doppler flow indexes methods and preliminary results. *American Journal of Obstetrics and Gynaecology*, **156**:1227–31.

Morris, P.J., Rennie, J.M., Evans, D.H. & Levene, M.I. (1989) Regional cerebral blood flow and Doppler flow velocity in the middle cerebral artery of the cat. *British Journal of Anaesthesia*, **63**:233p–234p

Muizelaar, J.P., Wei, E.P., Kontos, H.A. & Becker, D.P. (1986) Cerebral blood flow is regulated by changes in blood pressure and in blood viscosity alike. *Stroke*, **17**:44–8.

Mullaart, R.A., Hopman, J.C.W., De Haan, A.F.J., Rotteveel, J.J., Daniels, O. & Stoelinga, G.A.B. (1992) Cerebral blood flow fluctuations in low-risk preterm newborns. *Early Human Development* **30**:41–8.

Myers, T.F., Patrinos, M.E., Muraskas, J., Caldwell, C.C., Lambert, G.H. & Anderson, C.L. (1987) Dynamic trend monitoring of cerebral blood flow velocity in newborn infants. *Journal of Pediatrics*, **110**:611–16.

Newell, D.W., Aaslid, R., Stooss, R. & Reulen, H.J. (1992) The relationship of blood flow velocity fluctuations to intracranial pressure B waves. *Journal of Neurosurgery*, **76**:415–21.

Niijima, S., Shortland, D.B., Levene, M.I. & Evans, D.H. (1988) Transient hyperoxia and cerebral blood flow velocity in infants born prematurely and at full term. *Archives of Disease in Childhood*, **63**:1126–30.

Nishimaki, S., Yoda, H., Seki, K., Kawakami, T., Akamatsu, H. & Iwasaki, Y. (1990) Cerebral blood flow velocities in the anterior cerebral arteries and basilar artery in hydrocephalus before and after treatment. *Surgical Neurology*, **34**:373–4.

Panerai, R.P., Kelsall, A.W.R., Rennie, J.M. & Evans, D.H. (1995) Cerebral autoregulation dynamics in premature newborns. *Stroke*, **26**:74–80.

Perlman, J.M., Hill, A. & Volpe, J.J. (1981) The effect of patent ductus arteriosus on flow velocity in the anterior cerebral arteries ductal steal in the premature infant. *Journal of Pediatrics*, **99**:767–71.

Perlman, J.M. & Volpe, J.J. (1983) Seizures in the preterm infant: effects on cerebral blood flow velocity, intracranial pressure and arterial blood pressure. *Journal of Pediatrics*, **102**:288–93.

Perlman, J.M., McNenamin, J.B. & Volpe, J.J. (1983) Fluctuating cerebral blood flow velocity in respiratory distress syndrome. *New England Journal of Medicine*, **309**:204–9.

Pople, I.K., Quinn, M.W., Bayston, R. & Hayward, R.D. (1991) The Doppler pulsatility index as a screening test for blocked ventriculo-peritoneal shunts. *European Journal of Pediatric Surgery*, Suppl. 1:27–9.

Pryds, O., Greisen, G. & Johansen, K.H. (1988) Indomethacin and cerebral blood flow in preterm infants treated for patent ductus arteriosus. *European Journal of Pediatrics*, **147**:315–16.

Pryds, O., Greisen, G., Lou, H. & Friis-Hansen, B. (1989) Heterogeneity of cerebral vasorectivity in preterm infants supported by mechanical ventilation. *Journal of Pediatrics*, **115**:111–38.

Pryds, O., Anderson, G.E. & Friis-Hansen, B. (1990a) Cerebral blood flow reactivity in spontaneously breathing, preterm infants shortly after birth. *Acta Paediatrica Scandinavica*, **79**:391–6.

Pryds, O., Greisen, G., Lou, H. & Friis-Hansen, B. (1990b) Vasoparalysis associated with brain damage in asphyxiated term infants. *Journal of Pediatrics*, **117**: 119–25.

Pryds, O. & Schneider, S. (1991) Aminophylline reduces cerebral blood flow in stable preterm infants without affecting the visual evoked potential. *European Journal of Pediatrics*, **150**:366–9.

Quinn, M.W. Ando, Y. & Levene, M.I. (1992) Cerebral arterial and venous flow velocity measurements in post haemorrhagic ventricular dilatation and hydrocephalus. *Developmental Medicine and Child Neurology*, **34**:864–9.

Quinn, M.W. & Pople, I.K. (1992) Middle cerebral artery pulsatility in children with blocked cerebrospinal fluid shunts. *Journal of Neurology, Neurosurgery and Psychiatry*, **55**:325–7.

Raju, T.N.K., Go, M., Ryva J.C. & Schmidt, D.J. (1987) Common carotid artery flow velocity measurements in the newborn period with pulsed Doppler technique. *Biology of the Neonate* **32**:241–9.

Raju, T.N.K. & Zikos, E. (1987) Regional cerebral blood flow velocity in infants – a real time transcranial and fontanellar pulsed Doppler study. *Journal of Ultrasound in Medicine*, **6**:497–507.

Raju, T.N.K., Kim, S.Y. & Chapman, L. (1989) Circle of Willis flow patterns in healthy newborn infants. *Journal of Pediatrics*, **114**:455–8.

Ramaekers, V.Th., Casaer, P., Daniels, H., Smet, M. & Marchal, G. (1989) The influence of behavioural states on cerebral blood flow velocity in stable preterm infants. *Early Human Development*, **20**:229–46.

Ramaekers ,V.Th., Casaer, P., Daniels, H. & Marchal, G. (1992) The influence of blood transfusion on brain blood flow and autoregulation among stable preterm infants. *Early Human Development*, **30**:211–20.

Rennie, J.M., South, M. & Morley, C.J. (1987) Cerebral blood flow velocity variability in infants receiving artificial ventilation. *Archives of Disease in Childhood*, **62**:1247–51.

Rennie, J.M. (1989) Cerebral blood flow velocity variability after cardiovascular support in premature babies. *Archives of Disease in Childhood*, **64**:897–901.

Rennie, J.M., Morris, P.J., Evans, D.H., Levene, M.I. & Thoresen, M. (1990) Blood pressure exerts more influence on cerebral blood flow velocity than arterial carbon dioxide in piglets less than 24 hours old. *Early Human Development*, **21**:125.

Rennie, J.M., Coughtrey, H., Morley, R. & Evans, D.H. (1995) Comparison of cerebral blood flow velocity with cranial ultrasound imaging for early prediction of outcome in preterm infants. *Journal of Clinical Ultrasound*, **23**:27–31.

Rey, M., Segerer, H., Kiessling, C. & Obladen, M. (1994) Surfactant bolus instillation effects of different doses on blood pressure and cerebral blood flow velocities. *Biology of the Neonate*, **66**:16–21.

Rosenberg, A.A., Narayan, V. & Douglas Jones, M. (1985) Comparison of anterior cerebral artery blood flow velocity and cerebral blood flow during hypoxia. *Pediatric Research*, **19**:67–70.

Rosenkrantz, T.S. & Oh, W. (1984) Aminophylline reduces cerebral blood flow velocity in low birthweight infants. *American Journal of Diseases in Children*, **138**:489–91.

Rosenkrantz, T.S., Stonestreet, B.S., Hansen, N.B., Nowicki, P. & Oh, W. (1984) Cerebral blood flow in the newborn lamb with polycythaemia and hyperviscosity. *Journal of Pediatrics*, **104**:276–80.

Saliba, E., Chantepie, A., Marchand, M., Pourcelot, L. & Laugier, J. (1991) Intraoperative measurements of cerebral haemodynamics during ductus arteriosus ligation in preterm infants. *European Journal of Pediatrics*, **150**: 362–5.

Saliba, E., Autret, E., Nasr, C., Suc, A.L. & Laugier, J. (1992) Perinatal pharmacology and cerebral blood flow. *Biology of the Neonate* **62**:252–7.

Seibert, J.J., McCowan, T.C., Chadduck, W.M., Adametz, J.R., Glasier, C.M., Williamson, S.L., Taylor, B.J., Leithiser, R.E., McConnell, J.R., Stansell, C.A., Rodgers, A. & Corbitt, S.L. (1989) Duplex pulsed Doppler US versus intracranial pressure in the neonate: clinical and experimental studies. *Radiology*, **171**:155–9.

Shortland, D.B., Gibson, N.A., Levene, M.I., Archer, L.N.J., Evans, D.H. &

Shaw, D.E. (1990a) Patent ductus arteriosus and cerebral circulation in preterm infants. *Developmental Medicine and Child Neurology*, 32:386–93.

Shortland, DB., Levene, M.I., Archer, N., Shaw, D. & Evans, D.H. (1990b) Cerebral blood flow velocity recordings and the prediction of intracranial haemorrhage and ischaemia. *Journal of Perinatal Medicine*, 18:411–17.

Shuto, H., Yasuhara, A., Sugimoto, T., Iwase, S. & Kobayashi, Y. (1987) Longitudinal determination of cerebral blood flow velocity in neonates with the Doppler technique. *Neuropaediatrics*, 18:218–21.

Sonesson, S-E., Lundell, B.W.P. & Herin, P. (1986) Changes in intracranial blood flow velocities during surgical ligation of the patent ductus arteriosus. *Acta Paediatrica Scandinavica*, 75:36–42.

Sonesson, S-E., Winberg, P. & Lundell, B.W.P. (1987) Early postnatal changes in intracranial arterial blood flow velocities in term infants. *Pediatric Research*, 22:461–4.

Sonesson, S-E. & Herin, P. (1988) Intracranial arterial blood flow velocity and brain blood flow during hypocarbia and hypercarbia in newborn lambs: a validation of range-gated Doppler ultrasound flow velocimetry. *Pediatric Research*, 24:423–6.

Spencer, J.A.D., Giussani, D.A., Moore, P.J. & Hanson, M.A. (1991) In vitro validation of Doppler indices using blood and water. *Journal of Ultrasound in Medicine.* 10:305–8.

Strassburg, H.M., Bogner, K. & Klemm, H.J. (1988) Alterations of intracranial pressure and cerebral blood flow velocity in healthy neonates and their implication in the origin of perinatal brain damage. *European Journal of Pediatrics*, 147:30–5.

Task Force on Brain Death in Children (1987) Guidelines for the determination of brain death in children. *Pediatrics*, 80:298–300.

Thoresen, M., Haaland, K. & Steen, P.A. (1994) Cerebral Doppler and misrepresentation of flow changes. *Archives of Disease in Childhood*, 71:F103–F106.

Van Bel, F., Van de Bor, M., Buis-Liem, T.N., Stijnen, T., Baan, J. & Ruhy, J.H. (1987a) The relation between left-to-right shunt due to patent ductus arteriosus and cerebral blood flow velocity in preterm infants. *Journal of Cardiovascular Ultrasonography*, 6:19–25

Van Bel, F., Van de Bor, M., Stijnen, T., Baan, J. & Ruys, J.H. (1987b) Cerebral blood flow velocity patterns in healthy and asphyxiated newborns: a controlled study. *European Journal of Pediatrics*, 146: 461–7.

Van Bel, F., Van de Bor, M., Baan, J. & Ruys, J.H. (1988a) The influence of abnormal blood gases on cerebral blood flow velocity in the preterm newborn. *Neuropediatrics*, 19:27–32.

Van Bel, F., Van de Bor, M., Baan, J., Stijnen, T. & Ruys, J.H. (1988b) Blood flow velocity patterns of the anterior cerebral arteries. *Journal of Ultrasound in Medicine*, 7:553–9.

Van Bel, F., Den Ouden, L., Van de Bor, M., Baan, J. & Ruys, J.H. (1989a) Cerebral blood flow velocity during the first week of life of preterm infants and neurodevelopment at two years. *Developmental Medicine and Child Neurology*, 31:320–8.

Van Bel, F., Van de Bor, M., Stijnen, T., Baan, J. & Ruys, J.H. (1989b) Cerebral blood flow velocity changes after a single dose of indomethacin duration of its effects. *Pediatrics*, 84: 802–7.

Van Bel, F., Van de Bor, M., Stijnen, T., Baan, J. & Ruys, J .H. (1989c) Does caffeine affect cerebral blood flow in the preterm infant? *Acta Paediatrica Scandinavica*, 78:205–9.

Van Bel, F., De Winter, P.J., Wijnands, H.B.G., Van de Bor, M. & Egberts, J. (1992) Cerebral and aortic blood flow velocity patterns in preterm infants receiving prophylactic surfactant treatment. *Acta Paediatrica Scandinavica*, 81: 504–10.

Van De Bor, M. & Walther, F.J. (1991a) Cerebral blood flow velocity in healthy term infants. *American Journal of Medical Science*, 301:91–6.

Van de Bor, M. & Walther, F. (1991b) Cerebral blood flow velocity regulation in preterm infants. *Biology of the Neonate*, 59:329–35.

Van de Bor, M., Ma, E.J. & Walther, F.J. (1991) Cerebral blood flow velocity after surfactant instillation in preterm infants. *Journal of Pediatrics*, 118: 285–7.

Van Straaten, H.L.M., Rademaker, C.M.A. & De Vries, L.S. (1992) Comparison of the effect of midazolam or vecuronium on blood pressure and cerebral blood flow velocity in the premature newborn. *Developmental Pharmacology and Therapeutics*, 19:191–5.

Volpe, J.J., Herscovitch, P., Perlman, J.M. & Raichle, M.E. (1983) Positron emission tomography in the newborn. Extensive impairment of regional cerebral blood flow with intraventricular haemorrhage and haemorrhagic cerebral involvement. *Pediatrics*, 72:589–601.

Volpe, J.J. (1987) Brain death determination in the newborn. *Pediatrics*, 80:293–7.

Wilcox, W.D., Carrigan, T.A. & Dooley, K.J. (1983) Range-gated pulsed Doppler ultrasonographic evaluation of carotid arterial blood flow in small preterm infants with patent ductus arteriosus. *Journal of Pediatrics*, 102:294–8.

Winberg, P., Dahlstrom, A. & Lundell, B. (1986) Reproducibility of intracranial Doppler flow velocimetry. *Acta Paediatrica Scandinavica*, Suppl., 329:134–9.

Winberg, P., Sonesson, S-E. & Lundell, B. (1990) Postnatal changes in intracranial blood flow velocity in preterm infants. *Acta Paediatrica Scandinavica*, 79:1150–5.

Winkler, P. & Helmke, K. (1989) Duplex scanning of the deep venous drainage in the evaluation of blood flow velocity of the cerebral vascular system in infants. *Pediatric Radiology*, 19:79–90.

Wong, W.S., Tsruda, J.S., Liberman, R.L., Chirino, A., Vogt, J.F. & Gangitano, E. (1989) Color Doppler imaging of intracranial vessels in the neonate. *American Journal of Neuroradiology*, 10:425–30.

Wright, L.L., Baker, K., Hollander, D.I., Wright, J.N. & Nagey, D.A. (1988) Cerebral blood flow velocity in term newborn infants changes associated with ductal flow. *Journal of Pediatrics*, 112:768–73.

Yoshida, H., Yashura, A. & Kobayashi, Y. (1991) Transcranial Doppler sonographic studies of cerebral blood flow velocity in neonates. *Pediatric Neurology*, 7:105–10.

Yoshida-Shuto, H., Yashura, A. & Kobayashi, Y. (1992) Cerebral blood flow velocity and failure of autoregulatiin in neonates their relation to outcome of birth asphyxia. *Neuropaediatrics*, 23:241–4.

Zernikow, B., Michel, E., Kohlmann, G., Steck, J., Schmidtt, R.M. & Jorch, G. (1994) Cerebral autoregulation of preterm infants – a non-linear control system? *Archives of Disease in Childhood*, 71:F166–F173.

6 Vascular lesions I: lesions typical of mature infants

Introduction

In view of the importance and frequent occurrence of brain injury secondary to haemorrhage and ischaemia in preterm infants, a separate chapter has been devoted to these conditions. However, ultrasound diagnosis of many other vascular lesions is possible in both term and preterm infants, and these appearances are summarised here.

Postnatal consequences of fetal haemorrhage

In utero haemorrhage as a result of alloimmune thrombocytopaenia was described by Zalneraitis *et al.* in 1979. This condition remains the most likely cause of an intracranial haemorrhage present at birth in a term infant. Over 32 cases have now been reported with the earliest at 20 weeks gestation (De Vries *et al.*, 1988; Leidig *et al.*, 1988; Giovangrandi *et al.*, 1990; Govaert *et al.*, 1995). Antiplatelet antibodies were the cause of all the significant neonatal morbidity relating to neonatal thrombocytopaenia in a seven year prospective study enrolling over 15,000 women (Burrows & Kelton 1993). There were three cases of *in utero* intracranial haemorrhage amongst 18 affected pregnancies, one baby being stillborn. The frequency of human platelet antigen 1 (HPA1; formerly termed PLA$_1$) negative women in the Caucasian population is around 2.5%, with an expected birth prevalence of around 1 per 600. The fact that the observed incidence is lower than this probably results from a combination of under-diagnosis in mildly affected cases, and from the fact that the human leucocyte antigen (HLA) glycoproteins are expressed close to the HPA system on the platelet surface. HLA DRB3*0101 (HLA-DR52a) positive, HPA1 negative mothers are at increased risk (1:3) of developing alloimmunisation (Reznikoff-Etievant *et al* 1983). Figures 6.1(a) and (b) show the evolution of a parietal haemorrhage present at birth in a neonate with alloimmune thrombocytopaenia who was treated with washed maternal platelets and immunoglobulin (HPA1 negative donor platelets are now available). He was normal at 2 years. Figures 6.2(a) and (b) show a porencephalic cyst and ventriculomegaly present at birth in a similarly affected infant who developed progressive hydrocephalus.

Other coagulopathies such as factor V and factor VIII deficiency have been associated with *in utero* intracranial haemorrhage (Whitelaw *et al.*,

107

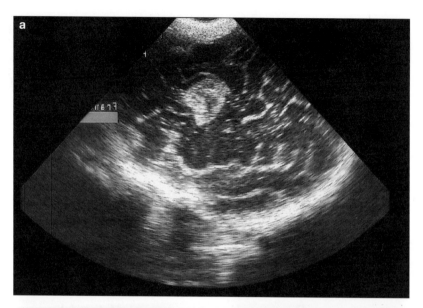

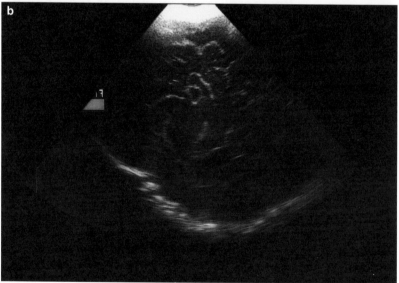

Fig. 6.1. *(a) Right tangential parasagittal appearance of a haemorrhage into the parietal lobe of a term infant suffering from alloimmune thrombocytopaenia. The echodense area is seen in the centre of the image. (b) The same anatomical site is occupied by a small dark, cystic area, which was taken two months later.*

1984; Schmid *et al.*, 1986), as has hydrops fetalis (Bose, 1978). Table 6.1 summarises the causes of prenatal intracranial lesions. Prenatal intracranial haemorrhage has caused congenital hydrocephalus (Jackson & Blumhagen, 1983; Mintz *et al.*, 1985; Leidig *et al.*, 1988). Prenatal haemorrhage was present in 2 of 59 fetuses with ventriculomegaly in a five-year series in

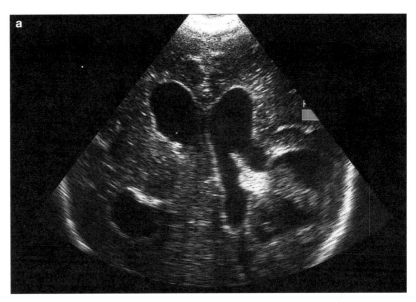

Fig. 6.2(a). *Coronal scan. The ventricles are large and on the left there is a poren-cephalic cyst in the temporal lobe. The dark cerebral spinal fluid containing space has an echo-reflectant area which is a clot.*

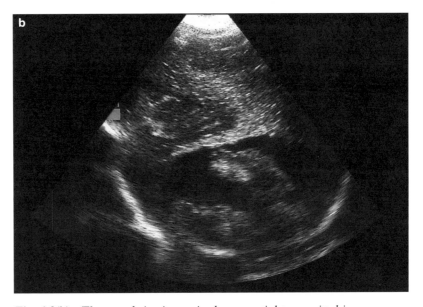

Fig. 6.2(b). *The same lesion is seen in the tangential parasagittal image.*

Table 6.1. *Causes of prenatal intracranial damage*

Coagulopathy secondary to alloimmune thrombocytopaenia
  secondary to hydrops fetalis
  secondary to factor V or factor VIII deficiency

Hypotension
  twin–twin transfusion syndrome
  maternal collapse (anaphylaxis, trauma, severe infection)

Infarction or thrombosis of arterial tree resulting in porencephalic cyst

Rupture of congenital cerebral arterio-venous malformation

Boston (Prober *et al.*, 1986). Twins are at eight times higher risk of cerebral palsy than singleton births and this risk increases to 1 in 100 when the co-twin has died in utero (Petterson *et al.*, 1993; Grether *et al.*, 1994; Szymonowicz *et al.*, 1986; Yoshioka *et al* 1979). White matter injury is thought to be sustained when the surviving twin experiences a period of hypotension because of acting as a pump twin during the agonal phase of his or her intrauterine partner (Fusi *et al.*, 1991). Maternal ill-health caused by anaphylactic shock, intercurrent infection or trauma has caused cerebral damage *in utero* (Erasmus *et al.*, 1982; Kim & Elyaderani, 1982; Stirling *et al.*, 1989). Arterio-venous malformations and congenital aneurysms can result in haemorrhage presenting in the perinatal period (Schum *et al.*, 1979; Lee *et al.*, 1978). Infarction of an artery, discussed later in this chapter, has also occurred in prenatal life.

Extracerebral haemorrhage

Subgaleal haemorrhage and cephalhaematoma

Figure 6.3 contains a diagrammatic key to the coverings of the brain and haemorrhage can occur at any level. The most superficial types of haemorrhage are difficult to detect with ultrasound, as is subarachnoid bleeding. Subgaleal haemorrhage is essentially a clinical diagnosis, and is an important condition because the loose nature of the tissue space can allow massive blood loss leading to shock. Babies develop boggy, diffuse swelling of the scalp. A clinical diagnosis of cephalhaematoma does not usually require investigation with ultrasound.

Subdural haemorrhage

Blood collects in the subdural space usually as a consequence of birth trauma, bleeding diathesis or rupture of a dural vascular malformation.

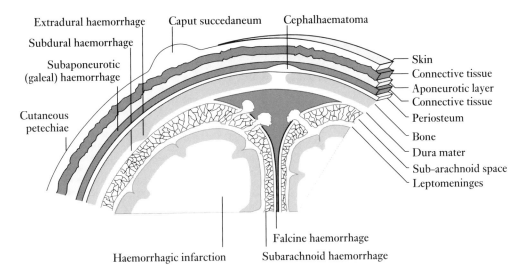

Fig. 6.3. *Diagram of the coverings of the brain.*

The condition often co-exists with hypoxic-ischaemic encephalopathy. Detection is important as drainage can reduce the risk of cerebral atrophy. Subdural bleeding may lead to occlusion of the arterial tree and vasospasm, producing an associated ischaemic lesion in the parenchyma of the brain. Figures 6.4(a–c) shows the appearance of subdural haemorrhage and associated infarction in the middle cerebral artery territory diagnosed with ultrasound in an infant delivered by Keilland's forceps who was carefully oberved because of fits, continuing hypotonia and an increasing fontanelle tension. Unfortunately the ultrasound diagnosis of subdural haemorrhage is not reliable, and it can be difficult to distinguish from a large subarachnoid collection or from external hydrocephalus caused by cerebral atrophy.

Growing skull fracture

This extremely rare condition, sometimes termed leptomeningeal cyst, requires the combination of two events: a dural tear and an underlying brain insult causing oedema. The swelling disrupts the dura at the time that repair should be taking place and as a consequence the fracture fails to heal, the bone edges deviate and eventually a pulsatile cerebrospinal fluid containing swelling appears on the surface of the skull. Figure 6.5(a) shows the appearance of the original parenchymal lesion in an infant under our care who developed a growing skull fracture as a result of damage to the dura below coronal suture during ventouse delivery (Fig. 6.5b). There was no skull fracture, and in this respect this case is almost identical to that of Hansen *et al.* (1987). Treatment required neurosurgical repair of the underlying dura, and was successful. The child was developing normally at one year.

111

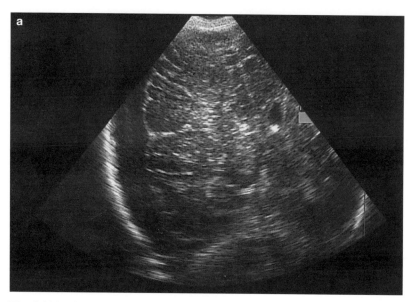

Fig. 6.4(a). *Coronal scan. There is midline shift to the left. A large echo-free zone is seen between the skull and the brain surface on the right. The parenchyma of the right side of the brain also appears more echo-reflectant ('bright') than usual, consistent with a vascular infarction.*

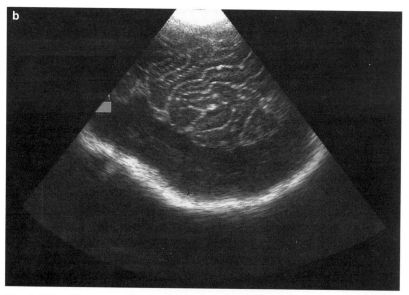

Fig. 6.4(b). *The appearances are confirmed in the tangential parasagittal image.*

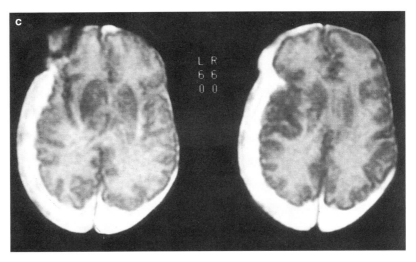

Fig. 6.4(c). *Magnetic resonance image corresponding to Figs. 6.4(a) and (b). The subdural collection appears as a white rim around the brain.*

Subarachnoid haemorrhage – generalised

This may give rise to an increased distance between the inner table of the skull and the surface of the brain as in Fig. 6.4, but a small subarachnoid bleed will not be detected by ultrasound. The distance between the lateral wall of the sagittal sinus and the surface of the brain was found to be about 2 mm in healthy term infants (Govaert *et al.*, 1989). Preterm infants normally have a larger gap between the inner table of the skull and the brain surface. Blood in the subarachnoid space can sometimes be seen filling the Sylvian fissure on a coronal view.

Focal subarachnoid haemorrhage (haematoma)

The ultrasound appearance of this condition was described as 'convexity cerebral haemorrhage' by Morgan *et al.* in 1983. Term infants, several of whom had required exchange transfusion for rhesus isoimmunisation were noted to have large echoreflectant areas, which at post-mortem were confirmed to be areas of haematoma into the subarachnoid space. Similar haemorrhage has resulted from alloimmune thrombocytopaenia and sepsis (Govaert, 1993). Haemostatic failure with disseminated intravascular coagulation resulting in focal subarachnoid bleeding has a predilection for the temporo-parietal convexity (Chessells & Wigglesworth 1970).

An example of this rare condition is shown in Fig. 6.6; this child had a third nerve palsy and was impaired at follow up. The midline shift suggests a subarachnoid origin of the bleeding rather than a haemorrhage into the temporal lobe. This would be the main differential diagnosis from the ultrasound appearance.

113

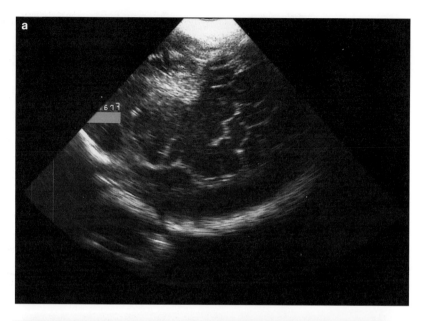

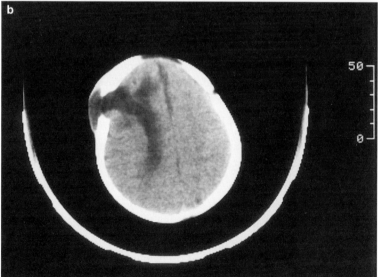

Fig. 6.5. *(a) A tangential parasagittal section of the brain showing a bright spot in the parietal cortex. In the computed tomography scan shown in (b) this area has become cystic and is continuous with a cerebral spinal fluid containing lesion on the skull surface, and the ventricular system. The areas are joined through a defect in the skull which occurred in the coronal suture line.*

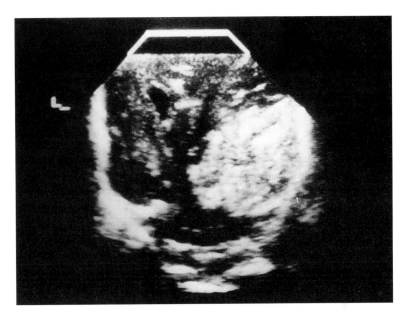

Fig. 6.6. *Large right convexity cerebral haemorrhage in a newborn suffering from rhesus isoimmunisation. The affected zone appears as a white patch in the temporal lobe.*

Bleeding into the falx and cavae

Bleeding into the falx is frequently described at post-mortem, but not often recognised in life. Haemorrhage into the cavum has been described using ultrasound (Butt *et al.*, 1985).

Intracerebral haemorrhage

Thalamic haemorrhage

Isolated thalamic bleeding can occur in term neonates without an associated intraventricular haemorrhage, whereas extension of intraventricular haemorrhage into the thalamus is often seen in preterm infants (Table 6.2). The underlying problem may be thrombosis of the internal cerebral vein (Govaert *et al.*, 1992). The infants present with seizures and may have eye signs including sunsetting, deviation and upgaze palsy although these are not universal (Trounce *et al.*, 1985; Montoya *et al.*, 1987; Roland *et al.*, 1990; De Vries *et al.*, 1992). The onset can be quite sudden with a bulging fontanelle, vomiting and jittering. Unilateral lesions have a better prognosis (De Vries *et al.*, 1992). Thalamic lesions have also been described in association with infection (Roland *et al.*, 1990; Weber *et al.*, 1992; Govaert *et al.*, 1992), coagulopathy and asphyxia (Kreusser *et al.*, 1984; Cabanas *et al.*, 1991). Appearances seen in infected babies include a striated pattern

115

Table 6.2. *Causes of thalamic lesions seen with ultrasound*

Isolated, cause unknown
Hypoxic ischaemic encephalopathy
Extension of intraventricular haemorrhage
Congenital infection such as toxoplasmosis
Acquired infection such as group B streptococcal sepsis
Coagulopathy secondary to polycythaemia or inherited disorder

probably due to vascular calcification (see Fig. 10.14 for an example). The baby whose scan is depicted in Fig. 6.7(a,b) was suffering from *Escherichia coli* meningitis. Recently magnetic resonance imaging has confirmed the previous pathological evidence that thalamic lesions occur very frequently after 'partial plus total' birth asphyxia and are not always haemorrhagic (Voit *et al.*, 1985; Rutherford *et al.*, 1994). Half the 17 cases described by Roland *et al.* (1990) were idiopathic.

Haemorrhagic arterial cerebral infarction

Neonatal strokes are rare, with an estimated incidence of 1 in 10,000 deliveries (Uvebrant, 1988). Arterial occlusion can result from an embolus, hyperviscosity, sepsis, stretching and damage to the artery from birth trauma or secondary to the oedema associated with birth asphyxia. Infants present with contralateral seizures. An ultrasound scan of the brain shows focal hyperdensity in the territory of the affected artery (Figs. 6.8a–b). Colour flow Doppler may demonstrate absence of arterial pulsations. CT scan shows a corresponding low-density area (Hill *et al.*, 1983). The right common carotid artery is sometimes ligated for vascular access in order to perform extracorporeal membrane oxygenation (ECMO), and this has caused several babies to develop areas of cerebral infarction (Schumacher *et al.*, 1988).

Intraventricular haemorrhage

This can occur in mature infants but as the appearances are identical to those in preterm infants this topic is not discussed separately here.

Cerebellar haemorrhage

Cerebellar bleeding is more common in the preterm than term infant, but the ultrasound scan appearances have been described and are the same in both groups (Reeder *et al.*, 1982). Scotti *et al.* (1981) drew attention to the poor prognosis.

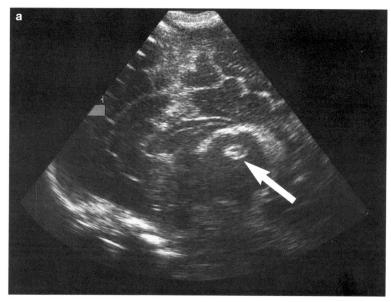

Fig. 6.7(a). *A parasagittal view in which there is a single small bright spot (arrowed) in the thalamus.*

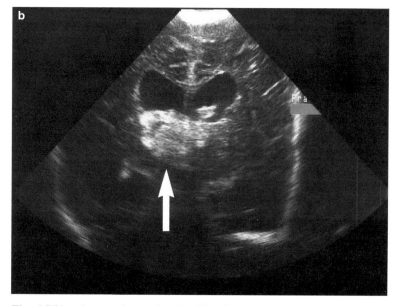

Fig. 6.7(b). *A coronal scan showing dilated ventricles and a haemorrhage into the right thalamus (arrowed), probably an extension from an intraventricular haemorrhage in this case.*

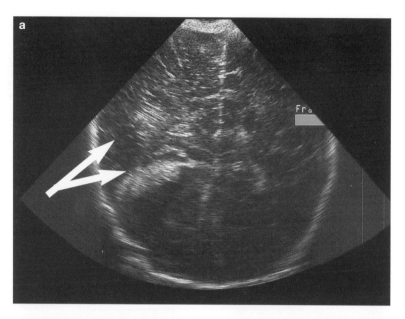

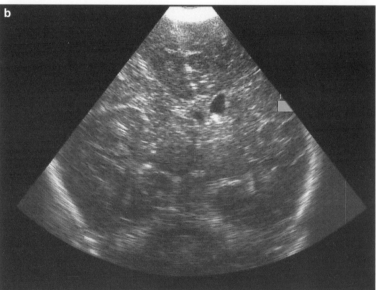

Fig. 6.8(a) and (b). *Two separate cases of coronal scans showing midline shift and focal hyperdensity in the region of the right middle cerebral artery (arrowed).*

Choroid plexus haemorrhage

The choroid often appears bright and bulky, particularly in preterm babies. A diagnosis of haemorrhage can be made if there is marked assymetry of the appearance of the choroid plexus together with an absence of intraventricular blood from an IVH. An example is given in Fig. 6.9(a–b). Bilateral

118

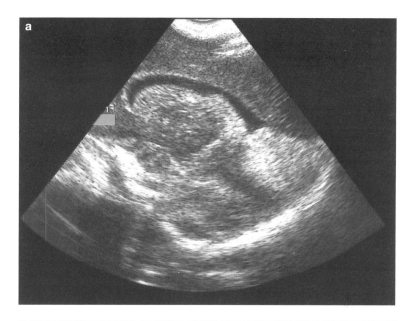

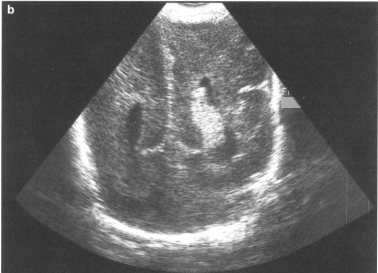

Fig. 6.9. *Parasagittal (a) and coronal (b) views showing asymmetrical bulk and brightness of the choroid plexus, situated in the trigone of the left ventricle.*

choroid plexus haemorrhage would be more difficult to diagnose and blood clot often settles around the choroid plexus in cases of intraventricular haemorrhage. The assumption that irregularity in the shape of the choroid plexus indicates haemorrhage is not correct.

References

Bose, C. (1978) Hydrops fetalis and *in utero* intracranial haemorrhage. Journal of Pediatrics, **93**:1023–4.

Burrows, R.F. & Kelton, J.G. (1993) Fetal thrombocytopaenia and its relation to maternal thrombocytopaenia. *New England Journal of Medicine*, **329**:1463–6.

Butt, W., Havill, D., Daneman, A. & Pape, K. (1985) Hemorrhage and cyst development in the cavum septi pellucidi and cavum vergae. *Pediatric Radiology*, **15**:368–71.

Cabañas, F., Pellicer, A., Perez-Higueras, A., Garcia-Alix, A., Roche, C. & Ouro, J. (1991) Ultrasonographic findings in thalamus and basal ganglia in term asphyxiated infants. *Pediatric Neurology*, **7**:211–15.

Chessells, J. M. & Wigglesworth, J. S. (1970) Secondary haemorrhagic disease of the newborn. *Archives of Disease in Childhood*, **45**:539–43.

De Vries, L.S., Connell, J., Bydder, G.M., Dubowitz, L.M.S., Rodeck, C.H., Mibashan, R.S. & Waters, A.H. (1988) Recurrent intracranial haemorrhage in *utero* in an infant with alloimmune thrombocytopaenia. *British Journal of Obstetrics and Gynaecology*, **95**:299–302.

De Vries, L.S., Smet, M., Goemans, W., Wilms, G., Devliger, H. & Casaer, P. (1992) Unilateral thalamic haemorrhage in the preterm and full term newborn. *Neuropediatrics*, **23**:153–6.

Erasmus, C., Blackwood, W. & Wilson, J. (1982) Infantile multicystic encephalomalacia after maternal bee-sting anaphylaxis during pregnancy. *Archives of Disease in Childhood*, **57**:785–7.

Fusi, L., McFarland, P., Fisk, N. & Wigglesworth, J.S., (1991) Acute twin-twin transfusion: a possible mechanism for brain-damaged survivors after intrauterine death of a monochorionic twin. *Obstetrics and Gynaecology*, **78**:517–20.

Giovangrandi, Y., Daffos, F., Kaplan, C., Forester, F. MacAleese, J. & Moirot, M. (1990) Very early intracranial haemorrhage in alloimmune fetal thrombocytopaenia. *Lancet*, **336**:310.

Govaert, P. (1993) Deep haemorrhage. In (ed. P. Govaert) *Cranial Haemorrhage in the Term Newborn Infant*, pp. 101–61. London: MacKeith Press.

Govaert, P., Pauwels, W., Vanhaesbrouck, P., De Praeter, C. & Afshrift, M. (1989) Ultrasound measurement of the subarachnoid space in infants. *European Journal of Pediatrics*, **148**:412–13.

Govaert, P., Achten, E., Vanhaesebrouck, P., De Praeter, C. & Van Damme, J. (1992) Deep cerebral venous thrombosis in thalamo-ventricular hemorrhage of the term newborn. *Pediatric Radiology*, **22**:123–127.

Govaert, P., Bridger, J. & Wigglesworth, J. (1995) Nature of the brain lesion in fetal neonatal alloimmune thrombocytopaenia. *Developmental Medicine and Child Neurology*, **37**:485–95.

Grether, J.K., Nelson, K.B. & Cummins, S.K. (1994) Twinning and cerebral palsy: experience in four northern California counties, births through 1983–1985. *Pediatrics*, 854–8.

Hansen, K.N., Pedersen, H. & Petersen, M.B. (1987) Growing skull fracture-rupture of coronal suture caused by vacuum extraction. *Neuroradiology*, **29**:502.

Hill, A., Martin, D.J., Daneman, A. & Fitz, C.R. (1983) Focal ischaemic cerebral injury in the newborn: diagnosis by ultrasound and correlation with computed tomographic scan. *Pediatrics*, **71**:790–3.

Jackson, J.C. & Blumhagen, J.D. (1983) Congenital hydrocephalus due to prenatal intracranial haemorrhage. *Pediatrics*, **72**:344–6.

Kim, M-S. & Elyaderani, M.K., (1982) Sonographic diagnosis of cerebroventricular haemorrhage *in utero. Radiology*, **142**:479–80.

Kreusser, K.L., Schmidt, R.E., Shackleford, G.D. & Volpe, J.J. (1984) Value of ultrasound for identification of acute haemorrhagic necrosis of thalamus and basal ganglia in an asphyxiated infant. *Annals of Neurology*, **16**:361–3.

Lee, Y.J., Kandall, S.R. & Ghali, V.S. (1978) Intracerebral arterial aneurysm in a newborn. *Archives of Neurology*, **35**:171–2.

Leidig, E., Dannecker, G., Pfeiffer, K.H., Salinas, R. & Peiffer, J. (1988) Intra-uterine development of posthaemorrhagic hydrocephalus. *European Journal of Pediatrics*, **147**:26–9.

Mintz, M.C., Arger, P.H. & Coleman, B.G. (1985) In-utero sonographic diagnosis of intracerebral haemorrhage. *Journal of Ultrasound in Medicine*, **4**:375–6.

Montoya, F., Couture, A., Frerebeau, P. & Bonnet, H. (1987) Hémorragie intraventriculaire chez le nouveau-né à terme: origine thalamique. *Pédiatrie*, **42**:205–9.

Morgan, M.E.I., Hensey, O.J. & Cooke, R.W.I. (1983) Convexity cerebral haemorrhage in the neonate: in vivo diagnosis. *Archives of Disease in Childhood*, **58**:814–8.

Petterson, B., Nelson, K.B., Watson, L. & Stanley, F. (1993) Twins, triplets and cerebral palsy in Western Australia in the 1980's. *British Medical Journal*, **307**: 1239–43.

Prober, B.R., Greene, M.F. & Holmes, L.B. (1986) Complexities of intraventricular abnormalities. *Journal of Pediatrics*, **108**: 545–51.

Reeder, J.D., Setzer, E.S. & Kaude, J.V. (1982) Ultrasonographic detection of perinatal intracerebellar hemorrhage. *Pediatrics*, **70**:385–6.

Reznikoff-Etievant, M.F., Muller, J.Y., Julien, F. & Paterau, C. (1981) HLA B8 and anti PLA 1 alloimmunization. *Tissue Antigens*, **18**:66–8.

Roland, E.H., Flodmark, O. & Hill, A. (1990) Thalamic haemorrhage with intraventricular haemorrhage in the full term newborn. *Pediatrics*, **85**:737–742.

Rutherford, M.A., Pennock, J.M. & Dubowitz, L.M.S. (1994) Cranial ultrasound and magnetic resonance imaging in hypoxic ischaemic encephalopathy: a comparison with outcome. *Developmental Medicine and Child Neurology*, **36**:813–25.

Schmid, G., Emons, D. & Kowalewski, S. (1986) Intracentrikuläre Hirnblutung des feten als Ursacke eines konnatalen Hydrozephalus. *Monatsschrift für Kinderheilkunde*, **134**:470–2.

Schum, T.R., Meyer, G.A., Grausz, J.P. & Glaspey, J.C. (1979) Neonatal intraventricular haemorrhage due to an intracranial arteriovenous malformation: a case report. *Pediatrics*, **64**:242–4.

Schumacher, R.E., Barks, J.D.E., Johnston, M.V., Donn, S.M., Scher, M.S., Roloff, D.W. & Bartlett, R.H. (1988) Right-sided brain lesions in infants following extracorporeal membrane oxygenation. *Pediatrics*, **82**:155–61.

Scotti, G., Flodmark, O., Harwood-Nash, D.C. & Humphries, R.P. (1981) Posterior fossa hemorrhages in the newborn. *Journal of Computer Assisted Tomography*, **5**:68–72.

Stirling, H.F., Hendry, M. & Brown, J.K. (1989) Prenatal intracranial haemorrhage. *Developmental Medicine and Child Neurology*, **31**:797–815.

Szymonowicz, W., Preston, H. & Yu, V.Y.H (1986) The surviving monozygotic twin. *Archives of Disease in Childhood*, **61**:454–8.

Trounce, J.Q., Fawer, C-L., Punt, J., Dodd, K.L., Fielder, A.R. & Levene, M.I. (1985) Primary thalamic haemorrhage in the newborn: a new clinical entity. *Lancet*, **i**:190–2.

Uvebrant, P. (1988) Hemiplegic cerebral palsy: aetiology and outcome. *Acta Paediatrica Scandinavica*, (Suppl.), 345.

Voit, T., Lemburg, P. & Stork, W. (1985) NMR studies in thalamic-striatal necrosis. *Lancet*, ii:445.

Weber, K., Riebel, Th. & Nasir, R. (1992) Hyperechoic lesions in the basal ganglia: an incidental finding in neonates and infants. *Pediatric Radiology*, 22:182–6.

Whitelaw, A., Haines, M.E., Bolsover, W. & Harris, E. (1984) Factor V deficiency and antenatal intracranial haemorrhage. *Archives of Disease in Childhood*, 59:997–9.

Yoshioka, H., Kadomoto, Y., Mino, M. Morikawa, Y., Kasubuchi, Y. & Kusunoki, T. (1979) Multicystic encephalomalacia in liveborn twin with a stillborn macerated co-twin. *Journal of Pediatrics*, 95:798–800.

Zalneraitis, E.L., Young, R.S.K. & Krishnamoorthy, K.S. (1979) Intracranial hemorrhage in utero as a complication of isoimmune thrombocytopenia. *Journal of Pediatrics* 95:611–14.

7 Vascular lesions II: lesions typical of immature infants

Haemorrhagic lesions of the preterm brain

History and terminology

Pathologists have recognised the existence of brain haemorrhage in infants since the nineteenth century, the first description of intraventricular haemorrhage being that of Cruveilhier in 1829 (Paneth *et al.*, 1994). A century later Ylppö (1919) documented the association with preterm birth, and Ruckensteiner & Zollner (1929) noted that the bleeding arose from the germinal matrix. Since the decline in subdural haemorrhage secondary to obstetric trauma bleeding into the germinal matrix or the lateral ventricle has become the most frequent form of intracranial haemorrhage in the neonatal period. 'Periventricular haemorrhage' has been widely used as a generic term, embracing germinal matrix haemorrhage, intraventricular haemorrhage and haemorrhage into the periventricular white matter. Direct extension into the parenchyma from pressure of blood in the ventricle is now considered unlikely. A better explanation for the frequent association of a unilateral parenchymal lesion with intraventricular haemorrhage is that the presence of a germinal matrix haemorrhage reduces the perfusion to the adjacent white matter by obstructing venous drainage. This type of parenchymal lesion, due to venous infarction, should be regarded as a complication of intraventricular haemorrhage (Gould *et al.*, 1987). Bleeding can also occur into areas of the brain previously rendered ischaemic (Rushton *et al.*, 1985). This condition, haemorrhagic periventricular leukomalacia, complicates about 15% of periventricular leukomalacia and is often bilateral (Armstrong & Norman, 1974). Although neuropathologically distinct, precise differentiation between types of parenchymal lesion in life using ultrasound is impossible. Some argue that all parenchymal lesions should be regarded as haemorrhagic periventricular leukomalacia (Guzzetta *et al.*, 1986). Levene has proposed the term germinal matrix haemorrhage-intraventricular haemorrhage (GMH-IVH) as the appropriate generic for the common form of intracranial haemorrhage seen in preterm infants (Levene & De Vries, 1995). Parenchymal lesions should be carefully described and photographed and not automatically assumed to be part of the 'periventricular haemorrhage' spectrum; this term, like those of 'Grade IV intraventricular haemorrhage' and 'parenchymal exten-

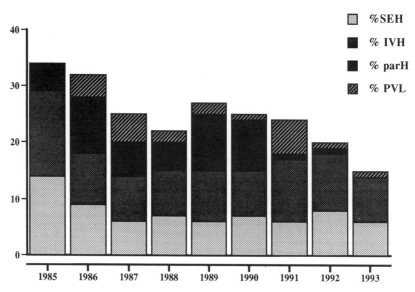

Fig. 7.1. *Incidence of brain injury by grade and year, Cambridge inborn very low birthweight infants (VLBWI) 1985–93. SEH: subependymal haemorrhage; IVH: intraventricular haemorrhage; parH: parenchymal haemorrhage; PVL: periventricular leukomalacia.*

sion of intraventricular haemorrhage' should be abandoned. In future other neuro-investigative techniques may allow differentiation of the types of parenchymal lesions during life.

Incidence and timing

Many cohort studies have been carried out to determine the incidence of GMH-IVH and parenchymal lesions in very low birthweight infants (<1500 g). In the early 1980s the incidence in this group was around 40% (Ahmann *et al.*, 1980; Dolfin *et al.*, 1983). Since then there has been a fall in incidence – Strand *et al.* (1990) reported a decrease from 30% to 24% between 1982 and 1985, Philip *et al.* (1989) a decrease from 39% to 25% between 1980 and 1987 and Szymonowicz *et al.* (1986b) from 40% to 25%. At the Rosie Maternity Hospital, Cambridge, UK (Fig. 7.1) we have documented a similar reduction in incidence from 35% to 15% since 1985. This trend to less severe bleeding and improved neuro-developmental outcome occurred in association with increased use of antentatal steroids (Rennie *et al.* 1996). A reduction has not been reported in all centres – the incidence of GMH-IVH and parenchymal lesions remained static in Liverpool between 1980 and 1989 (Cooke, 1991). All forms of GMH-IVH are more common in very premature babies (Fig. 7.2 a). The association between gestational age and periventricular leukomalacia is much weaker (Fig. 7.2b).

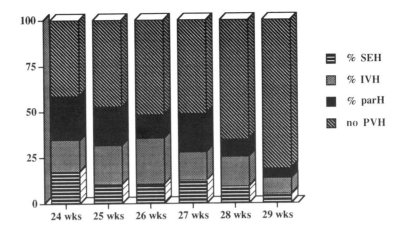

Fig. 7.2(a). *Incidence of GMH–IVH (germinal matrix haemorrhage–intraven-tricular haemorrhage) and parenchymal lesions by gestational age, Cambridge. SEH: subependymal haemorrhage; IVH: intraventricular haemorrhage; parH: parenchymal haemorrhage; PVH: periventricular haemorrhage.*

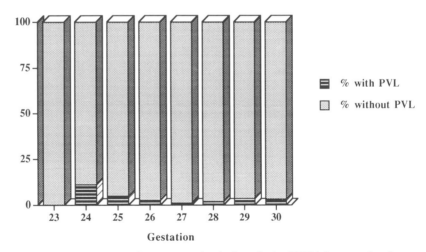

Fig. 7.2(b). *Incidence of periventricular leukomalacia (PVL) by gestational age, Cambridge.*

There is a consensus that in three-quarters of cases GMH-IVH has occurred by 72 hours of postnatal age (Dolfin *et al.*, 1983; Szymono-wicz & Yu., 1984). In 10–20% of cases further progression takes place over the next 24–48 hours (Levene & De Vries, 1984). The optimal time to perform a single sonogram to screen for GMH-IVH in very low birthweight infants is therefore 4–7 days after birth (Partridge *et al.*, 1983), although many neonatal units have the facility to perform more frequent scans and carry out an initial examination within 24 hours after birth. Leviton and co-workers (1988, 1991) have suggested several times that very early GMH-IVH might have a different aetiology, and this plausible hypothesis remains to be further explored. GMH-IVH of prenatal onset has been described (Leech & Kohnen 1974). Repeat scans at 14 days and before discharge are required to detect periventricular leukomalacia.

Aetiology and prevention

The main factors which predispose to GMH-IVH are prematurity and the presence of respiratory distress syndrome. Within this group of sick preterm infants many variables have been examined and it is difficult to extract those which may be causal from those which are merely associates. The best unifying hypothesis is that GMH-IVH occurs because of a combination of haemodynamic instability together with a propensity to bleed which is intrinsic to the newborn. Change in cerebral blood flow can occur in sick infants as a result of hypercarbia, hypoglycaemia or hypoxia. Changes in the systemic blood pressure are more likely to be transmitted to the cerebral circulation if autoregulation is disturbed. Rapid alteration in blood pressure occurs with handling, suction, drug therapy and artificial ventilation. The preterm infant is more likely to suffer haemorrhage resulting from a pre-existing coagulation defect; the balance of prostaglandin synthesis is shifted towards anticoagulation and the neonatal platelet has a storage pool defect. Twelve specific agents have been used as prophylaxis against GMH-IVH in very low birthweight infants, but none has gained general acceptance. The best advice is to offer a high standard of intensive care, particularly in the vital first few hours; this may mean antenatal transfer to a tertiary centre, and certainly should include consideration of antenatal steroid therapy. Phenobarbitone and vitamin K have also been given to mothers expected to deliver prematurely, with some success (Shankaran *et al.*, 1986; Morales *et al.*, 1988). There is no convincing evidence that the mode of delivery can affect the incidence of GMH-IVH, but bruising and asphyxia should be avoided. Stabilisation of blood gases, blood pressure and temperature together with the administration of surfactant and an attempt to avoid the baby fighting the ventilator are far more important than the administration of a drug, particularly in a unit where the incidence of GMH-IVH is known to be less than 20% (Szymonowicz *et al.*, 1986b). Gentle handling, limiting suction, avoiding twisting the baby's neck and preventing rapid infusions of colloid and bicarbonate unless shock is present are also helpful (Kling, 1989).

Accuracy of ultrasound diagnosis

In spite of the widespread use of ultrasound diagnosis of GMH-IVH for audit and research, suprisingly little work has been done on autopsy verification of ultrasound findings. Paneth *et al.* (1994) found the sensitivity for detection of lesions <0.2 cm was poor, with only 29% being diagnosed, although this increased to 50% when the child survived long enough to have three or more scans. Larger haemorrhages, more than 1 cm diameter, were all identified. Hope *et al.* (1988) studied 56 cases and reported a sensitivity and specificity of 61 and 78% for germinal matrix haemorrhage; 91 and 81% for intraventricular haemorrhage. The large number of false positive and negative diagnoses for small (<0.5cm) germinal matrix haemorrhage has also been noted by others (Thorburn *et al.*, 1982; Trounce *et al.*, 1986a; Carson *et al.*, 1990). Corbett *et al.* (1991) assessed intra-observer and inter-observer reliability amongst radiologists used to interpreting cranial ultrasound scans and found excellent agreement only when a basic classification system (normal/abnormal) was used.

Classification

The original classification system suggested by Papile in 1978 was based on computerised tomographic scan diagnosis of GMH-IVH. She proposed four grades of severity: (I) where haemorrhage was confined to the germinal matrix, (II) where blood was present in the ventricular cavity but not distending it, (III) where the ventricular cavity was enlarged and full of blood and (IV) where there was bleeding into the parenchyma of the brain. This classification system has the merit of simplicity and was quickly adapted for ultrasound diagnosis of GMH-IVH, although concern has been raised regarding the difficulty of distinguishing grades II and III – it has been pointed out that all infants with IVH eventually develop a degree of ventricular enlargement (Flodmark *et al.*, 1980). McMenamin *et al.* (1984) suggested a classification based on mild (subependymal), moderate (intermediate amount of blood in enlarged ventricle) or severe (haemorrhage filling and enlarging ventricle forming a cast and/or intracerebral extension). With the increasing realisation that all parenchymal echodense lesions are not necessarily part of the same disease alternative systems have been proposed. Levene & De Crespigny (1983) suggested that the presence of haemorrhage should be coded as H with subscripts of 0–4, ventricular dilatation as V with degrees of severity, and parenchymal lesions as P also with three grades (Table 7.1). A normal scan would be coded as H_0, V_0. Even this complex system fails to fully account for periventricular leukomalacia and no classification system has become internationally accepted. The prognosis depends on the initial and final ultrasound appearances which may evolve over time. Numerical systems without firm agreed definitions can only be confusing and I suggest describing the appearances as either germinal matrix haemorrhage or intraventricular haemorrhage; if the ventricle appears enlarged, it is best to measure it (Chapter 8). Parenchymal lesions should be carefully described and permanently recorded as previously discussed.

127

Table 7.1. *The classification system of Levene & De Crespigny (1983)*

Grade	Description
Haemorrhage	
H_0	No haemorrhage
H_1	Localised haemorrhage <1cm maximum
H_2	Haemorrhage >1cm but not extending beyond the atrium
H_3	Blood clot forming a cast of the ventricle
H_4	Intraparenchymal haemorrhage
Ventricular dilatation	
V_0	No dilatation
V_1	Transient dilatation
V_2	Persistent but stable dilatation requiring treatment
V_3	Progressive dilation requiring treatment
V_4	Persistent asymmetrical dilatation
Parenchymal	
P_1	Porencephalic cyst in communication with the ventricle
P_2	Intraparenchymal cyst separated from the ventricle by ependyma
P_3	Intraparenchymal haemorrhage separate from the ventricle

Description of the ultrasound appearances of periventricular haemorrhage

Germinal matrix haemorrhage (subependymal haemorrhage)

In this type of intracranial haemorrhage, bleeding is confined to the germinal matrix capillary bed. Pathological studies indicate that bleeding starts in the outer region of the matrix, not the region bordering the ventricle (Paneth *et al.*, 1994). The most frequent position for bleeding to occur is in the caudothalamic groove at the head of the caudate nucleus, although bleeding can occur into germinal matrix tissue in the temporal or occipital sites (Fig. 7.3). The germinal matrix structure is unique to the preterm infant and regresses after 32 weeks gestation, partly explaining the rarity of the condition in mature infants. Eventually the haemorrhage is replaced by a cavity, seen on ultrasound as a small subependymal cyst, which is of remarkably little consequence considering the importance of the glia that were destroyed. Germinal layer haemorrhage thus resolves over a period of weeks. Pathological studies reveal invasion of haemosiderin-laden macrophages and repeated ultrasonography can show a echodense line which probably reflects this (Fig. 7.4).

Ultrasound diagnosis rests on the demonstration, in two planes, of an echogenic area at the head of the caudate nucleus. The most important distinction to be made is from the normal choroid plexus which tucks into

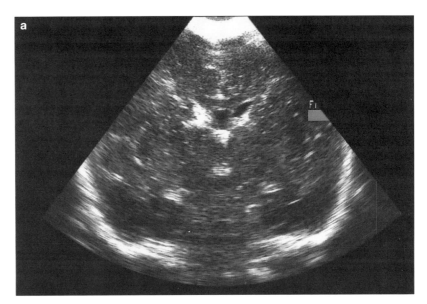

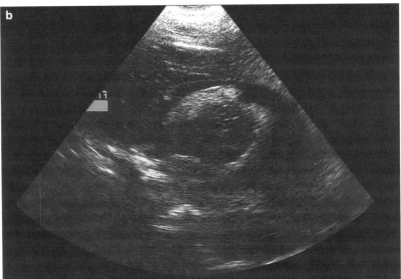

Fig. 7.3. *Germinal matrix haemorrhage seen in coronal (a) and parasagittal view (b).*

the thalamocortical groove. To be certain that a germinal matrix haemorrhage exists it must be clearly separate from the choroid plexus. Assymetry can help in difficult decisions.

Intraventricular haemorrhage

A germinal layer haemorrhage may rupture through the overlying ependyma, filling the ventricular system with blood (Fig. 7.5). Intraventricular

129

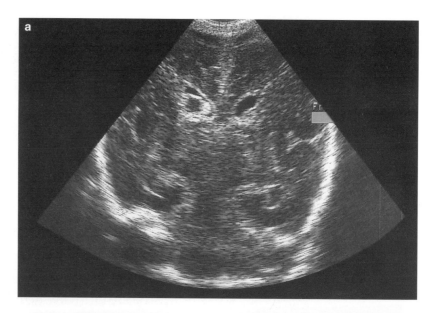

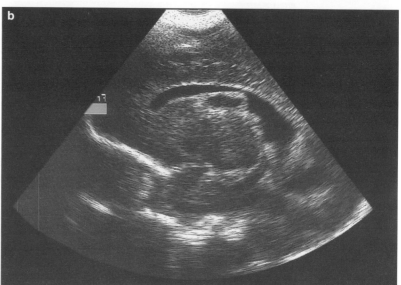

Fig. 7.4. *Resolving germinal matrix haemorrhage forming a subependymal cyst seen in coronal (a) and parasagittal (b) views. Note the white line around the perimeter of the ventricle, which may be due to haemosiderin deposition.*

haemorrhage may also arise from choroid plexus bleeding. The blood clot appears bright, and may form a cast of the ventricular system, distending it beyond the normal size (Fig. 7.6). Cast formation is almost universally followed by ventriculomegaly, which in half the cases progresses to hydro-cephalus.

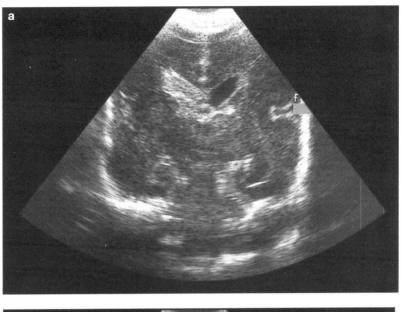

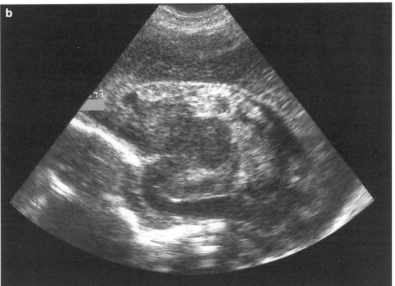

Fig. 7.5. *Intraventricular haemorrhage seen in coronal (a) and parasagittal (b) views.*

Parenchymal lesions

It is impossible to reliably distinguish haemorrhagic periventricular leuko-malacia from a primary parenchymal haemorrhage, white matter gliosis or infarction (Carson *et al.*, 1990). Features suggesting an ischaemic aetiology include the apex of the triangle of echodensity sitting at the lateral border

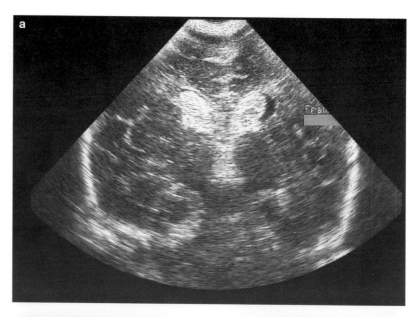

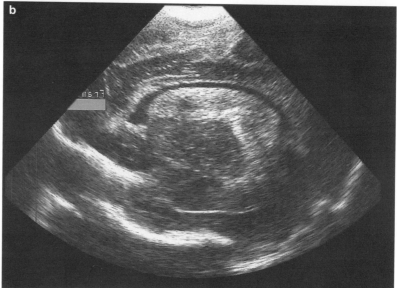

Fig. 7.6. *A large intraventricular haemorrhage seen in coronal (a) and parasagittal (b) sections. There is blood in the third ventricle visible in (a).*

of the ventricle rather than in the midline, a fluffy 'cotton wool' appearance to the outside margins and final evolution to multiple cysts which are not in communication with the ventricle. Parenchymal haemorrhage associated with intraventricular haemorrhage tends to be unilateral and to evolve into a single porencephalic cyst which is in communication with the ventricle. The early appearance is that of a bright, clearly defined echodensity with

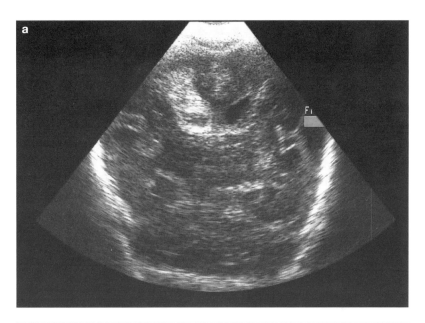

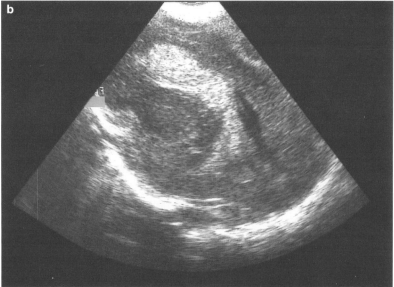

Fig. 7.7. *Parenchymal lesion probably occurring as a complication of GMH–IVH (germinal matrix haemorrhage–intraventricular haemorrhage), which is present on the right side. (a) Coronal view; (b) parasagittal view.*

the apex of the triangle in the midline and a smooth outer margin (Fig. 7.7). Later a large cyst develops, often with a clot attached to the wall (Fig. 7.8). Pathological appearances are shown in Fig. 7.9. A porencephalic cyst (Fig. 7.10) is usually followed by a hemiplegia, which does not impair

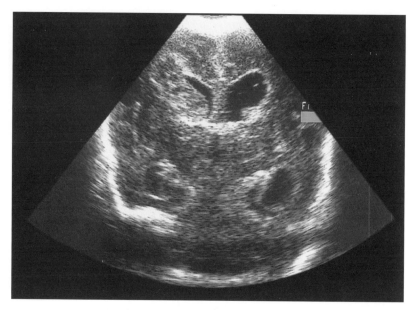

Fig. 7.8. *Evolution of the lesion seen in Fig. 7.7 after 12 days. There is ventriculo-megaly. The parenchymal lesion is becoming echolucent and a large cyst is forming.*

the intellect, whereas multiple cystic periventricular leukomalacia presages spastic diplegia often accompanied by developmental delay.

Ischaemic lesions of the preterm brain; periventricular leukomalacia

History and terminology

For over a century, periventricular leukomalacia has been described in the brains of infants dying in the neonatal period, and the fact that the condition was more common in preterm infants was ascribed to increased vulnerability of immature white matter. The term periventricular leukomalacia (literally: white matter softening) was introduced by Banker and Larroche in their study of 51 cases, published in 1962. That the lesions apparently occurred in a boundary zone between a ventriculofugal and ventriculopetal circulation was suggested by Takashima & Tanaka (1978). The vascular boundary zone hypothesis is the current favourite with most authors, and is supported by several of the aetiological factors, although the presence of the requisite arterial pattern has been disputed (Kuban & Gilles, 1985). Hypoperfusion is unlikely to be the sole cause, and toxins or excitatory amino acids may play a role in reducing local blood and energy supply.

Incidence and timing

There are far fewer reliable cohort studies of preterm infants reporting the incidence of periventricular leukomalacia than for GMH-IVH. Compari-

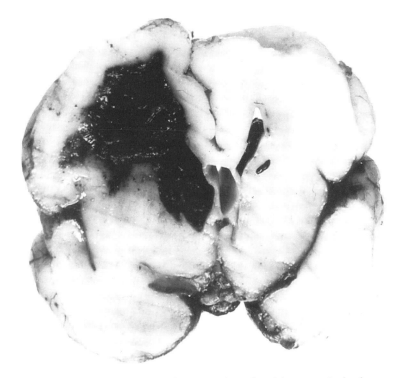

Fig. 7.9. *Pathological specimen with a parenchymal and intraventricular haemorrhage.*

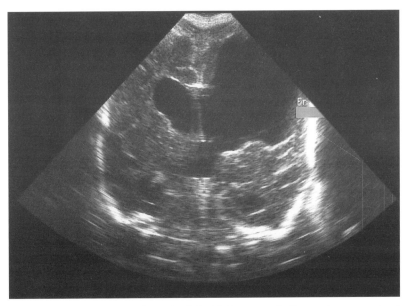

Fig. 7.10. *A massive, single cavity left-sided porencephalic cyst in communication with the ventricle.*

sons are also more difficult because the definition varies, and because periventricular leukomalacia can develop at up to 40 weeks postconceptual age. The reported incidence thus varies according to the number of ultrasound scans performed, the definition and the resolving power of the transducer used. De Vries & Levene (1995) summarise the published reports which vary from 2–3% (Calvert *et al.*, 1986; De Vries *et al.*, 1988 a–c) to 17.8% (Sinha *et al.*, 1985). At the Rosie Maternity Hospital, Cambridge, UK the incidence of cystic periventricular leukomalacia is about 2% amongst inborn very low birthweight infants (Fig. 7.2b).

In contrast to GMH-IVH, which occurs within the first week, periventricular leukomalacia has been reported to develop up to 11 weeks after birth. The areas of increased echodensity which precede the cystic lesions appear within 24–48 hours of the insult, the cysts evolving 2–4 weeks later. The median time to cyst development was 21 days in one study (Trounce *et al.*, 1986b). The cysts remain visible for several weeks but eventually disappear leaving glial scars or generalised cerebral atrophy.

Aetiology and prevention

Prematurity is not such a clear risk factor for periventricular leukomalacia as it is for GMH-IVH (De Vries *et al.*, 1988c; Ikonen *et al.*, 1988). Antepartum factors are more important in periventricular leukomalacia than for GMH-IVH and the condition has been described after antepartum haemorrhage, after maternal anaphylaxis due to bee-stings or intravenous iron and after maternal road traffic accidents (Spinillo *et al.*, 1993; Sinha *et al.*, 1985; Weindling *et al.*, 1985). Doppler studies of the fetus which demonstrate reversed umbilical arterial flow at end-diastole, have been followed by the development of parenchymal lesions in postnatal life in some studies but not others (Karsdorp *et al.*, 1994; Scherjon *et al.*, 1993). Monochorial twin pregnancy, particularly where there is death of the co-twin, can result in antenatal white matter necrosis (Bejar *et al.*, 1988, 1990). Szymonowicz *et al.* (1986a) found that in 56 cases of surviving monozygotic twins, 76% had a cerebral lesion. Chorioamnionitis appeared to be a risk factor (Bejar *et al.*, 1988), as was acidosis after delivery (Low *et al.*, 1990).

After birth there have been associations reported with hypotension requiring inotropic support (De Vries *et al.*, 1988c; Iida *et al.*, 1992), hyperbilirubinaemia (Ikonen *et al.*, 1988, 1992) and necrotising enterocolitis particularly requiring surgery (Trounce *et al.*, 1988). Further indirect support for an ischaemic aetiology comes from the observation that reverse flow in the major cerebral arteries associated with patent ductus may be a risk factor (Sinha *et al.*, 1985; Shortland *et al.*, 1990). Hypocarbia from over enthusiastic artificial ventilation may predispose to periventricular leukomalacia (Calvert *et al.*, 1987; Ikonen *et al.*, 1992; Fujimoto *et al.*, 1994). Other implicated complications of prematurity include apnoea, hyperbilirubinaemia and infection (Ikonen *et al.*, 1988; De Vries & Levene, 1995). The obervation that the condition appeared more common in babies who had been multiply transfused (Sinha *et al.*, 1985) led to the suggestion

Table 7.2. *Classification of periventricular leukomalacia (PVL) based on cranial ultrasound appearances (De Vries* et al. *1992)*

Grade of PVL	Description
Grade I	Periventricular echodense area, persistent for seven days or more
Grade II	Periventricular echodense areas evolving into localised small fontoparietal cysts
Grade III	Periventricular echodense areas evolving into multiple cysts in the parieto-occipital white matter
Grade IV	Echodense areas in the deep white matter evolving into multiple subcortical cysts (multicystic encephalopathy)

that free radical injury might be important. A single oral dose of allopurinol failed to reduce the incidence of periventricular leukomalacia in a large randomised trial (Russell & Cooke, 1995).

Diagnosis and classification of periventricular leukomalacia

There is less experience with the ultrasound diagnosis of periventricular leukomalacia than GMH-IVH because the high frequency transducers required to visualise small cysts were not available until the mid-1980s. The first descriptions of the ultrasound appearances were those of Hill *et al.* (1982) and Levene *et al.* (1983). The realisation that echodense lesions in the parenchyma are not always part of the spectrum of GMH-IVH means that earlier studies must be interpreted with caution. There is as yet no generally accepted grading system for periventricular leukomalacia, but the one suggested by De Vries (Table 7.2) is easy to remember and apply (De Vries *et al.*, 1992; De Vries & Levene, 1995). One disadvantage of this system is that with experience it is possible to distinguish degrees of extent and severity within Grade 1 (Figs. 7.11–7.14) but this is not of practical importance unless the baby dies; significant 'flares' always become cystic if the baby survives. Pidcock *et al.* (1990) proposed that the term 'severe echodensity' should be reserved for a lesion that extended into the brain for a distance exceeding twice that of the ventricles on a coronal scan. The other drawback of this grading system is that it does not take into account the size of the cysts, which should be recorded together with the permanent record of the image.

Ultrasound diagnosis of periventricular leukomalacia

Grade I and II: periventricular 'flares' disappearing or evolving into small cysts

Serial ultrasonography reveals areas of increased echodensity which precede cystic periventricular leukomalacia in many cases (Figs. 7.11–7.14).

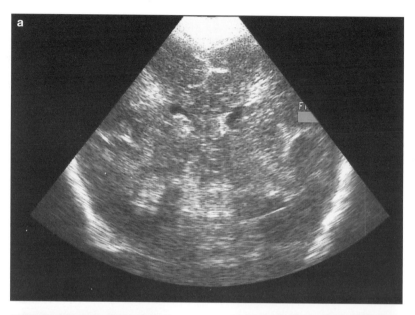

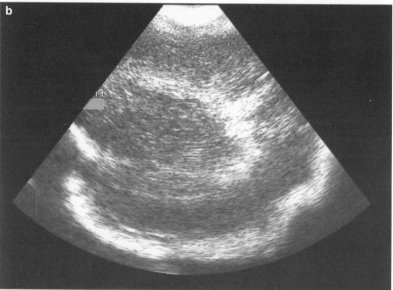

Fig. 7.11. *Periventricular echodensity present in the coronal (a) and parasagittal (b) views. The echodensity is as bright as the temporal bone, but is not very extensive and might resolve.*

Periventricular echodensities can disappear without subsequent cystic change. Post mortem correlations are few, but it has been shown that the 'flare' corresponds to areas of necrosis of the premyelin cells with a glial cell inflammatory response, although Hope reported a high false negative detection rate for gliosis with ultrasound (Hope *et al.*, 1988). In cases

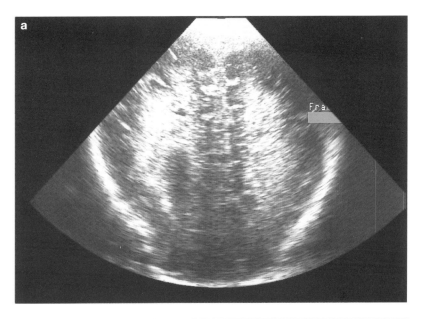

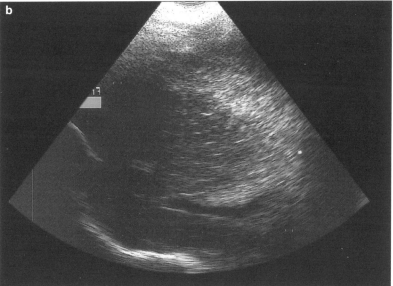

Fig. 7.12. *Marked periventricular echodensity in the occipital region seen on coronal (a) and parasagittal (b) scans. Small cysts are already developing on the right side in (a).*

where a flare appears after an acute collapse the ultrasound changes occur after 24–48 hours (Fig. 7.14). The degree of brightness of the echodense area distinguishes these lesions from the normal periventricular 'blush' described in Chapter 3, and most neonatal ultrasonographers would not classify a case as exhibiting a definite 'flare' unless the appearances were

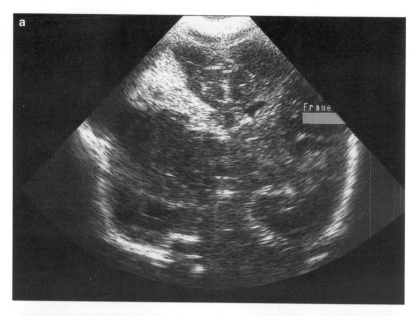

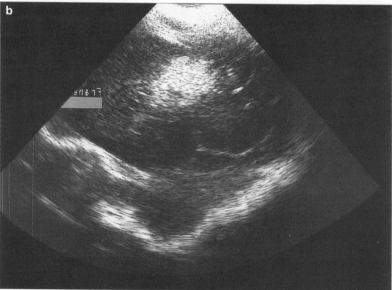

Fig. 7.13. *Further examples of periventricular echodensity which is probably ischaemic: (a) is a coronal and (b) a parasagittal section.*

apparent in both the parasagittal and coronal plane and persisted for more than 48 hours. Trounce *et al.* (1986b) only classified cases as 'prolonged flare' if the signs persisted for two weeks: De Vries *et al.*, (1992) suggest a week. Half of the 'flares' disappear within 10 days, and only about 10% evolve into small cysts after 2–4 weeks. These appearances represent the milder end of the spectrum of leukomalacia and can be followed by normal

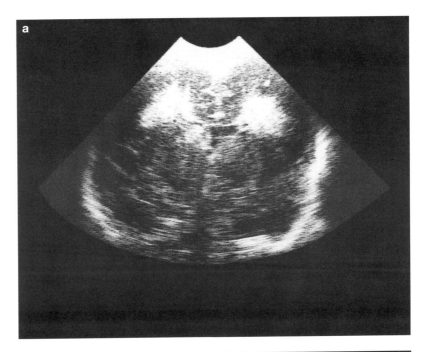

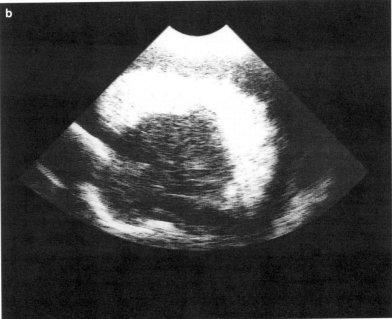

Fig. 7.14. *A very marked extensive bilateral periventricular echodensity. The apex of the triangles are at the ventricular border (unlike that in Fig. 7.7) and there is no associated GMH–IVH (germinal matrix haemorrhage–intraventricular haemorrhage). The apperances occurred 24 hours after an episode of ventricular fibrillation. The coronal section is shown in (a) and the parasagittal section in (b).*

141

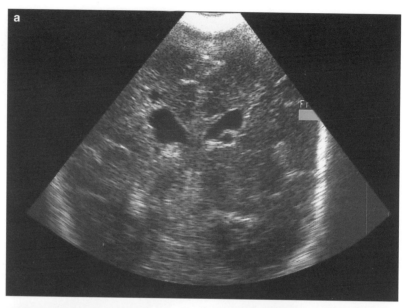

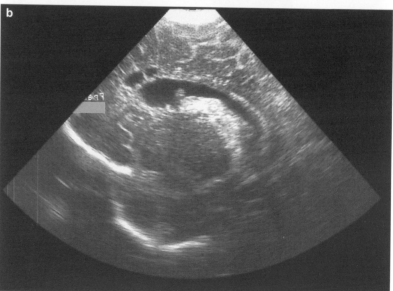

Fig. 7.15. *Small (< 1 cm) cysts in the periventricular zone seen on the right in the coronal section (a) and in the frontal region in the parasagittal view (b).*

development or transient dystonia (Chapter 12). Whether these mild lesions will reliably predict neurological abnormalities and cerebral dysfunction in later childhood remains to be seen. The area may be replaced by a glial scar, more often there is delayed myelination and ventricular dilatation (De Vries *et al.*, 1988c).

142

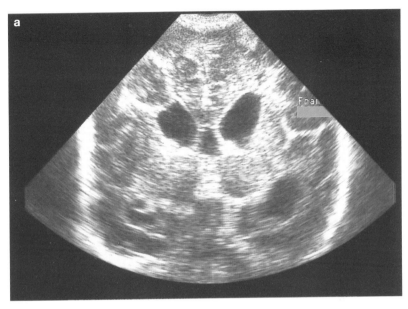

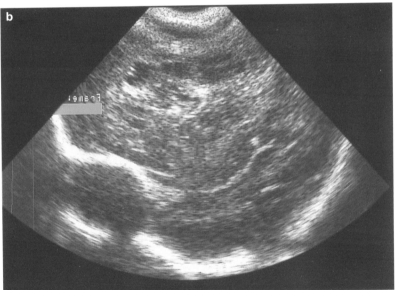

Fig. 7.16. *Mid-zone cystic periventricular leukomalacia in coronal (a) and parasagittal (b) section.*

Grade III: multiple cysts in the white matter

Multiple cysts of periventricular leukomalacia are a rare finding in preterm infants, occuring in about 2% of infants with birthweight below 1500g (Trounce *et al.*, 1986b; Calvert *et al.*, 1986; Sinha *et al.*, 1985). Their presence is a marker of a poor neurological prognosis, as almost all the

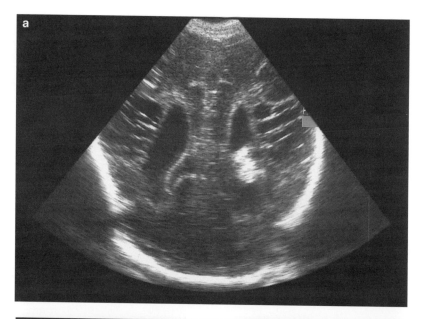

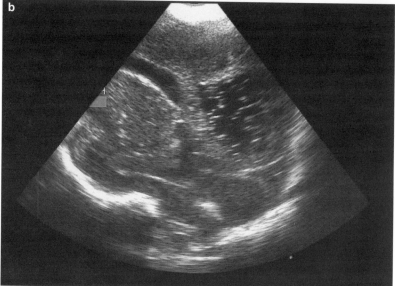

Fig. 7.17(a) and (b). *Massive bilateral occipital parenchymal cysts which developed in a child who had been hydropic* in utero.

children who have been followed up have developed cerebral palsy (Chapter 12). Figure 7.15 shows small anterior cysts, Fig. 7.16 more extensive mid-zone change and Fig. 7.17 extensive bilateral occipital cysts. The child whose scan appears as Fig. 7.16 (b) was growth retarded with reverse end-diastolic flow seen on Doppler studies of the umbilical artery. Bilateral occipital cysts greater than 1 cm in diameter, as seen in Fig. 7.17, carry the worst prognosis. The sensitivity and specificity between

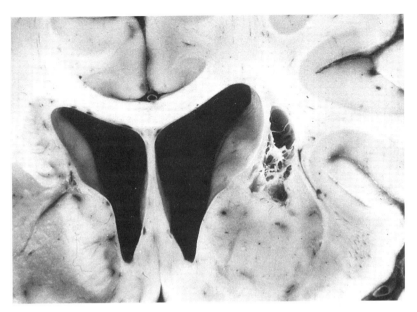

Fig. 7.18. *Small cystic lesions in the periventricular white matter seen at post-mortem.*

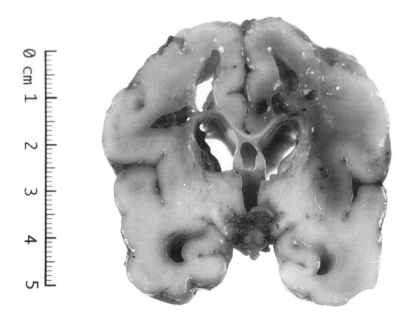

Fig. 7.19. *White matter softening and cystic change seen at post-mortem.*

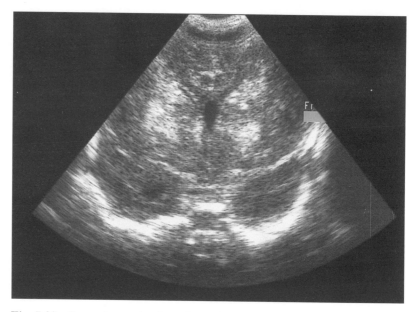

Fig. 7.20. *Coronal scan showing echodensity in the thalamic regions.*

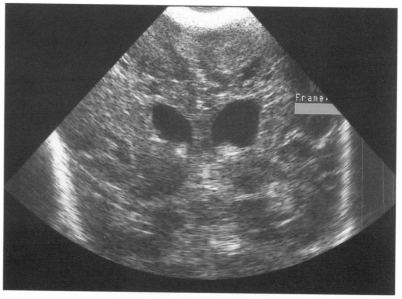

Fig. 7.21. *Subcortical leukomalacia developing in the same infant seen in Fig. 7.20.*

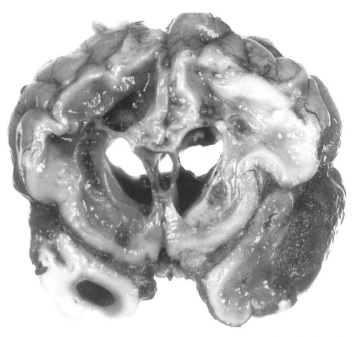

Fig. 7.22. *Pathological specimen showing extensive subcortical cystic change.*

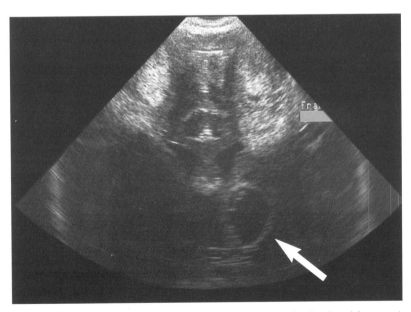

Fig. 7.23. *Wedge-shaped echodensity in a term infant who developed hypotension secondary to a pericardial effusion. A thalamic cyst (arrow) is also present.*

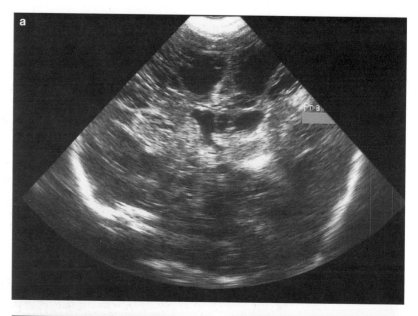

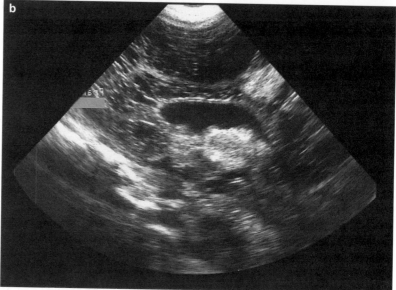

Fig. 7.24. *Coronal (a) and parasagittal (b) appearance of extensive subcortical cystic leucomalacia which developed in a term infant after an APH (antepartum haemorrhage).*

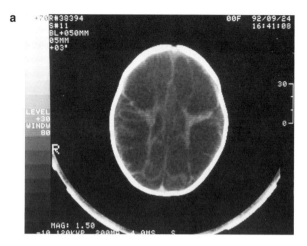

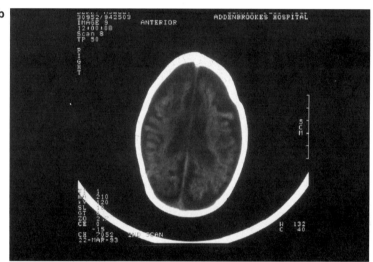

Fig. 7.25. *Computed tomography scan in the same infant as in Fig. 7.24, showing early (a) and late (b) appearances.*

ultrasound and post-mortem for the detection of small cysts is good (Fawer *et al.*, 1985; Trounce *et al.*, 1986b). Figures 7.18 and 7.19 are pathological specimens with cystic periventricular leukomalacia.

Grade IV: subcortical cysts or multicystic encephalopathy

This very severe form of white matter injury is more typical of hypoxic-ischaemic damage in the term infant. Figure 7.20 shows the appearances seen on a coronal scan immediately after birth in a preterm infant who was delivered prematurely because of growth retardation and Doppler evidence of reversed flow in the umbilical artery. The initial appearances show bright thalami and slit-like ventricles and these evolved to ventriculo–

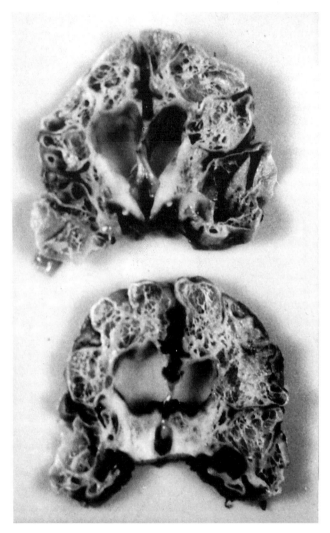

Fig. 7.26. *Pathological specimen of a brain like that seen in Fig. 7.24.*

megaly and cystic change over the next week (Fig. 7.21). Post mortem revealed extensive white matter injury (Fig. 7.22). Massive echodensity extending from the subcortical region to the periventricular zone is seen in Fig. 7.23, a scan performed in an infant who developed hypotension secondary to a pericardial effusion after a liver transplant. A thalamic cyst can also be seen on the left side (arrowed). Extensive subcortical leukomalacia in a term infant who had sustained perinatal asphyxia after a massive antepartum haemorrhage suffered by her mother at home is seen in Fig. 7.24. A CT scan showed the extent of lost neural tissue (Fig. 7.25), and later ultrasound scans revealed the formation of external hydrocephalus after involution of the cortex. Cysts formed in the subcortical region tend to be larger than those seen in grades II and III periventricular leukomalacia and they persist much longer. Figure 7.26 shows a brain affected by severe multicystic periventricular leukomalacia.

References

Ahmann, P.A., Lazzara, A., Dykes, F.D., Brann, J.F. & Schwartz, J.F. (1980) Intraventricular haemorrhage in the high risk preterm infant: incidence and outcome. *Annals of Neurology*, **7**:118–24.

Armstrong, D. & Norman, M.G. (1974) Periventricular leukomalacia in neonates: complications and sequelae. *Archives of Disease in Childhood*, **49**:367–75.

Banker, B.Q. & Larroche, J-C. (1962) Periventricular leukomalacia of infancy: a form of neonatal hypoxic encephalopathy. *Archives of Neurology*, **7**:386–410.

Bejar, R., Wosniak, P., Allard, M., Benirshke, K., Vaucher, Y, Coen, R., Berry, C., Schragg, P., Villegas, I. & Resnik, R. (1988) Antenatal origin of neurologic damage in newborn infants. I. Preterm infants. *American Journal of Obstetrics and Gynaecology*, **159**:357–63.

Bejar, R., Vigliocco, G., Gramajo, H., Solana, C., Bernischke, K., Berry, C., Coen, R. & Resnik, R. (1990)) Antenatal origin of neurologic damage in newborn infants. II. Multiple gestations. *American Journal of Obstetrics and Gynaecology*, **162**:1230–6.

Calvert, S.A., Hoskins, E.M., Fong, K.W. & Forsyth, S.C. (1986) Periventricular leukomalacia: ultrasonic diagnosis and neurological outcome. *Acta Paediatrica Scandinavica*, **75**:489–96.

Calvert, S.A., Hoskins, E.M. & Fong, K.W. (1987) Etiological factors associated with the development of periventricular leukomalacia. *Acta Paediatrica Scandinavica*, **76**:254–9.

Carson, S.C., Hertzberg, B.S., Bowie, J.D. & Burger, P.C. (1990) Value of sonography in the diagnosis of intracranial haemorrhage and periventricular leukomalacia: a postmortem study of 35 cases. *American Journal of Radiology*, **155**:595–601.

Cooke, R.W.I. (1991) Trends in preterm survival and incidence of cerebral haemorrhage 1980–1989. *Archives of Disease in Childhood*, **66**:403–7.

Corbett, S.S., Rosenfeld, C.R., Laptook, A.R., Risser, R., Maravilla, A.M., Dowling, S. & Lasky, R. (1991) Intraobserver and interobserver reliability in assessment of neonatal cranial ultrasound scans. *Early Human Development*, **27**:9–17.

De Vries, L.S., Regev, R., Pennock, J.M. Wiggelsworth, J.S. & Dubowitz, L.M.S. (1988a) Ultrasound evolution and later outcome of infants with periventricular densities. *Early Human Development*, **16**:225–3.

De Vries, L.S., Regev, R., Dubowitz, L.M.S., Whitelaw, A. & Aber, V.R. (1988b) Perinatal risk factors for the development of extensive cystic leukomalacia. *American Journal of Disease in Childhood*, **142**:732–5.

De Vries, L.S., Wigglesworth, J.S., Regev, R. & Dubowitz, L.M.S. (1988c) Evolution of periventricular leukomalacia during the neonatal period and infancy: correlation of imaging and postmortem findings. *Early Human Development*, **17**:205–19.

De Vries, L.S., Eken, P. & Dubowitz, L.M.S. (1992) The spectrum of leukomalacia using cranial ultrasound. *Behavioural Brain Research*, **49**:1–6.

De Vries, L.S. & Levene, M.I. (1995) Cerebral ischaemic lesions. In: *Fetal and Neonatal Neurology and Neurosurgery* ed. M.I. Levene & R.J. Lilford, pp. 267–86. Churchill Livingstone: Edinburgh.

Dolfin, T., Skidmore, M.B., Fong, K.W., Hoskins, E.M. & Shennan, A.T. (1983) Incidence, severity and timing of subependymal and intraventricular haemorrhages in preterm infants born in a perinatal unit as detected by serial real-time ultrasound. *Pediatrics*, **71**:541–6.

Fawer, C.L., Calame, A., Perentes, E. & Anderegg, A. (1985) Periventricular leukomalacia: a correlation study between real-time ultrasound and autopsy findings. *Neuroradiology*, **27**:292–300.

Flodmark, O., Fitz, C.R. & Harwood-Nash, D.C. (1980) CT diagnosis and short-term prognosis of intracranial hemorrhage and hypoxic-ischaemic brain damage in neonates. *Journal of Computer Assisted Tomography*, **5**:663–73.

Fujimoto, S., Togari, H., Yamaguchi, N., Mizutani, F., Suzuki, S. & Sobajima, H. (1994) Hypocarbia and cystic periventricular leukomalacia in preterm infants. *Archives of Disease in Childhood*, **71**:F107–F110.

Gould, S.J, Howard, S., Hope, P.L. & Reynolds, E.O.R. (1987) Periventricular intraparenchymal cerebral haemorrhage in preterm infants: role of venous infarction. *Journal of Pathology*, **151**:197–202.

Guzzetta, F., Shackleford, G.D., Volpe, S., Perlman, J.M. & Volpe, J.J. (1986) Perinventricular intraparenchymal echodensities in the newborn: critical determinants of neurologic outcome. *Pediatrics*, **78**:995–1006.

Hill, A., Melson, L., Clark, H.B. & Volpe, J.J. (1982) Haemorrhagic periventricular leukomalacia: diagnosis by real time ultrasound and correlation with autopsy findings. *Pediatrics*, **69**:282–4.

Hope, P.J., Gould, S.J., Howard, S., Hamilton, P.A., Costello, A.M. de L. & Reynolds, E.O.R. (1988) Precision of ultrasound diagnosis of pathologically verified lesions in the brains of very preterm infants. *Developmental Medicine and Child Neurology*, **30**:457–71.

Iida, K., Takashima, S. & Takeuchi Y. (1992) Etiologies and distribution of neonatal leukomalacia. *Pediatric Neurology*, **8**:205–9.

Ikonen, R.S., Kuusinen, E.J., Janas, M.O., Koivikko, M.J. & Sorto, A.E. (1988) Possible etiological factors in extensive periventricular leukomalacia of preterm infants. *Acta Paediatrica Scandinavica*, **77**:489–95.

Ikonen, R.S., Janas, M.O., Koivikko, M.J., Laippala, P. & Kuusinen, E.J. (1992) Hyperbilirubinaemia, hypocarbia and periventricular leukomalacia in preterm infants: relationship to cerebral palsy. *Acta Paediatrica Scandinavica*, **81**:802–7.

Karsdorp, V.H.M, van Vugt, J.M.G., van Geijn, H.P., Lostense, P.J., Arduini, D., Montenegro, N. & Todros, T. (1994) Clinical significance of absent or reversed end diastolic velocity waveforms in umbilical artery. *Lancet*, **344**: 1664–8.

Kling, P. (1989) Nursing interventions to decrease the risk of periventricular intraventricular haemorrhage. *Journal of Obstetric, Gynaecological and Neonatal Nursing*, 457–64.

Kuban, K.C.K. & Gilles, F.H. (1985) Human telencephalic angiogenesis. *Annals of Neurology*, **17**:539–48.

Leech, R.W. & Kohnen, P. (1974) Subependymal and intraventricular haemorrhages in the newborn. *American Journal of Pathology*, **77**:465–75.

Levene, M.I. & De Crespigny, L. Ch., (1983) Classification of intraventricular haemorrhage. *Lancet* i: 643.

Levene, M.I., Wigglesworth, J.S. & Dobowitz, V. (1983) Haemorrhagic periventricular leukomalacia in the neonate: a real time ultrasound study. *Pediatrics*, **71**:794–7.

152

Levene, M.I. & De Vries, L.S. (1984) Extension of neonatal intraventricular haemorrhage. *Archives of Disease in Childhood*, **57**:631–6.

Levene, M.I. & De Vries, L.S. (1995) Neonatal intracranial haemorrhage. In *Fetal and Neonatal Neurology and Neurosurgery*, ed. M.I. Levene & R.J. Lilford, pp. 335–66. Churchill Livingstone, Edinburgh.

Leviton, A., Pagano, M. & Kuban, K.C.K. (1988) Etiologic heterogeneity of intracranial haemorrhage in preterm newborns. *Pediatric Neurology*, **4**:274–8.

Leviton, A., Pagano, M., Kuban, K.C.K., Krishnamoorthy, K.S., Sullivan, K.F. & Allred, E.N. (1991) The epidemiology of germinal matrix hemorrahge during the first half-day of life. *Developmental Medicine and Child Neurology*, **33**:138–45.

Low, J.A., Froese, A.F., Galbraith, R.S., Sauerbrei, E.E, McKinven, J.P. & Karchmer, E.J. (1990) The association of fetal and newborn metabolic acidosis with severe periventricular leukomalacia in preterm newborns. *American Journal of Obstetrics and Gynaecology*, **162**:977–82.

McMenamin, J.B., Shackleford, G.D. & Volpe, J.J. (1984) Outcome of neonatal intraventricular hemorrhage with periventricular echodense lesions. *Annals of Neurology*, **15**:285–90.

Morales, W.J., Angel, J.L, O'Brien, W.F., Knuppel, R.A. & Marsalisi, F. (1988) The use of antenatal vitamin K in the prevention of early neonatal intraventricular haemorrhage. *American Journal of Obstetrics and Gynecology*, **159**:774–9.

Paneth, N., Rudelli, R., Kazam, E. & Monte, W. (1994) Brain damage in the preterm infant. *Clinics in Developmental Medicine*, No 131. Lavenham: Mac-Keith Press.

Papile, L-A., Burstein, J., Burstein, R. & Koffler, H. (1978) Incidence and evolution of subependymal and intraventricular hemorrhage: a study of infants with birthweight <1500g. *Journal of Pediatrics*, **92**:529–34.

Partridge, J.C., Babcock, D.S., Steichen, J.J. & Han, B.K. (1983) Optimal timing for diagnostic cranial ultrasound in low birth weight infants: detection of intracranial hemorrhage and ventricular dilatation. *Journal of Pediatrics*, **102**:281–7.

Philip, A.G.S., Allan, W.C., Tito, A.M. & Wheeler, L.R. (1989) Intraventricular hemorrhage in preterm infants: declining incidence in the 1980s. *Pediatrics*, **84**:797–801.

Pidcock, F.S., Graziani, L.J., Stanley, C., Mitchell, D.G. & Merton, D. (1990) Neurosonographic features of periventricular echodensities associated with cerebral palsy in preterm infants. *Journal of Pediatrics* **116**:417–22.

Rennie, J.M., Wheater, M. & Cole, T.J. (1996) Antenatal steroid administration is associated with an improved chance of intact survival in preterm infants. *European Journal of Paediatrics.* **155**: 576–9.

Ruckensteiner, E. & Zollner, F. (1929) Uber die Blutungen im Gebiete der Vena terminais bei Neugeborenen. *Frankfurt Zeitschrift für Pathologie*, **37**:568–78.

Rushton, D.I., Preston, P.R. & Durbin, G.M. (1985) Structure and evolution of echodense lesions in the neonatal brain: a combined ultrasound and necropsy study. *Archives of Disease in Childhood*, **60**:798–808.

Russell, G. & Cooke R.W.I. (1995) Randomised controlled trial of allopurinol prophylaxis in very preterm infants. *Archives of Disease in Childhood*, **73**:F27–F31.

Scherjon, S.A., Smolders-DeHaas, H., Kok, J.H. & Zonervan, H.A. (1993) The 'brain-sparing' effect: antenatal cerebral Doppler findings in relation to neurologic outcome in very preterm infants. *American Journal of Obstetrics and Gynaecology*, **169**:169–75.

Shankaran, S., Cepeda, E.E., Ilgan, N., Mariona, F., Hassan, M., Bhatia, R.,

Ostrea, E., Bedard, M.P. & Poland, R.L. (1986) Antenatal phenobarbital for the prevention of neonatal intraventricular haemorrhage. *American Journal of Obstetrics and Gynecology*, **154**:53–7.

Shortland, D.B., Gibson, N.A., Levene, M.I., Archer, L.N.J., Evans, D.H. & Shaw, D.E. (1990) Patent ductus arteriosus and cerebral circulation in preterm infants. *Developmental Medicine and Child Neurology*, **32**:386–93.

Sinha, S.K., Davis, J.M., Sims, D.G. & Chiswick, M.L. (1985) Relation between periventricular haemorrhage and ischaemic brain lesions diagnosed by ultrasound in very preterm infants. *Lancet*, **ii**:1154–5.

Spinillo, A., Fazzi, E., Stronati, M., Ometto, A., Iasci, A. & Guaschino, S. (1993) Severity of abruptio placentae and neurodevelopmental outcome in low birthweight infants. *Early Human Development*, **35**:45–54.

Strand, C., Laptook, A.R., Dowling, S., Cambell, N., Lasky, R.E., Wallin, L.A., Maravilla, A.M. & Rosenfeld, C.R. (1990) Neonatal intracranial hemorrhage: I. Changing pattern in inborn low-birth-weight infants. *Early Human Development*, **23**:117–28.

Szymonowicz, W. & Yu, V.Y.H. (1984) Timing and evolution of periventricular haemorrhage in infants weighing less than 1250 g at birth. *Archives of Disease in Childhood*, **59**:7–12.

Szymonowicz, W., Preston, H. & Yu, V.Y.H. (1986a) The surviving monozygotic twin. *Archives of Disease in Childhood*, **61**:454–8.

Szymonowicz, W., Yu, V.Y.H., Walker, A. & Wilson, F. (1986b) Reduction in periventricular haemorrhage in preterm infants. *Archives of Disease in Childhood*, **61**:661–5.

Takashima. J. & Tanaka, K. (1978) Development of cerebral architecture and its relationship to periventricular leukomalacia. *Archives of Neurology*, **35**:11–16.

Thorburn, R.J., Lipscomb, A.P., Reynolds, E.O.R., Blackwell, R.J., Cusick, G., Shaw, D.G. & Smith, J.F. (1982) Accuracy of imaging of the brains of newborn infants by linear-array real time ultrasound. *Early Human Development*, **6**:31–46.

Trounce, J.Q., Fagan, D. & Levene, M.I. (1986a) Intraventricular haemorrhage and periventricular leukomalacia in the preterm neonate: ultrasound and autopsy correlation. *Archives of Disease in Childhood*, **62**:1203–7.

Trounce, J.Q., Rutter, N. & Levene, M.I. (1986b) Periventricular leukomalacia and intraventricular haemorrhage in the preterm neonate. *Archives of Disease in Childhood*, **61**:1196–202.

Trounce, J.Q., Shaw, O.E., Levene, M.I. & Rutter, N. (1988) Clinical risk factors and periventricular leukomalacia. *Archives of Disease in Childhood*, **63**:17–22.

Weindling, A.M., Wilkinson, A.R., Cook, J., Calvert, S.A., Fok, T.-F. & Rochefort, M.J. (1985) Perinatal events which precede periventricular haemorrhage and leukomalacia in the newborn. *British Journal of Obstetrics and Gynaecology*, **92**:1218–23

Ylppö, A. (1919) Pathologisch-anatomische Studien bei Fruhgeborenen. *Zeitschrift fur Kinderheilkunde*, **20**:212–431.

8 *Enlarged cerebral ventricles*

Introduction

Ultrasound is the investigation of first choice for an infant with a large head, and may quickly identify both enlarged ventricles and the underlying cause. A normal result can provide equally rapid reassurance, and if the child is asymptomatic without clinical signs of raised intracranial pressure no further investigation is usually required. Ventriculomegaly in very low birthweight infants is often discovered during routine imaging, before the head enlarges. For monitoring the progress of ventricular enlargement and the response to treatment of hydrocephalus in infancy, ultrasound imaging is the method of choice. To facilitate this, several measurement systems have been devised, of which the best validated and most widely used is the ventricular index of Levene (1981).

Cause of ventriculomegaly: cerebral atrophy versus hydrocephalus

Large lateral ventricles can be caused by raised intracranial pressure due to overproduction of cerebrospinal fluid, an obstruction to its normal circulation or a failure of reabsorption. The ventricular system may enlarge without raised pressure; this is sometimes termed 'normal pressure hydrocephalus' and is a consequence of reduced cerebral substance (Hill & Volpe, 1981). The distinction between ventricular dilatation due to cerebral atrophy from that secondary to raised intracranial pressure is the key to correct diagnosis and management of a newborn with ventriculomegaly. Cerebral atrophy tends to be associated with irregularly shaped ventricles and there may be evidence of loss of white matter in the parenchyma with cysts of periventricular leukomalacia. Periventricular leukomalacia and GMH-IVH can co-exist, however, so that the existence of cysts does not mean that the ventriculomegaly is certain to be due to atrophy.

Extensive cerebral atrophy can cause the brain to shrink away from the inside of the skull leaving a gap. This is termed 'external hydrocephalus' (Fig. 8.1), and can further confuse the picture as the ventricular cavity can then be quite small. External hydrocephalus is difficult to detect with ultrasound. In cerebral atrophy head growth is normal or reduced, the fontanelle is lax and there are no symptoms of raised intracranial pressure.

155

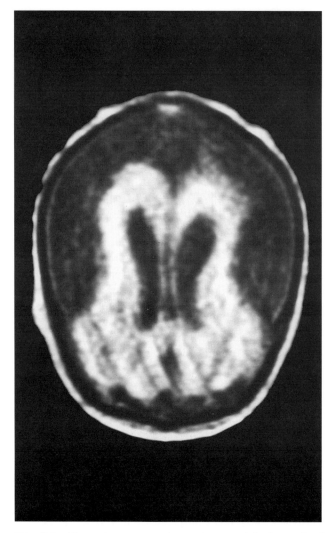

Fig. 8.1. *Magnetic resonance image in an axial plane, showing external hydro-cephalus. The brain has shrunk away from inside the skull leaving a rim of fluid.*

Progressive hydrocephalus tends to begin with trigonal (occipital horn) enlargement and is associated with increased occipitofrontal circumference, a tense fontanelle and separation of the sutures. The cerebrospinal fluid pressure is raised, usually above 10 cm, although hydrocephalus can be slowly progressive in preterm infants with a cerebrospinal fluid pressure within the normal range (up to 7.8 cm cerebrospinal fluid, Kaiser & Whitelaw, 1985). Symptoms of raised intracranial pressure include apnoea, convulsions, irritability, poor feeding and vomiting. Clinical signs are sunsetting of the eyes, bulging fontanelle and dilated scalp veins. Sunsetting refers to a visible rim of conjunctiva above the coloured iris and the eyelid.

Ventriculomegaly may be congenital or acquired, and the diagnosis can

Table 8.1. *Causes of hydrocephalus and cerebral atrophy classified by age at onset*

Congenital hydrocephalus
  Aqueduct stenosis
  Dandy-Walker malformation
  Arnold Chiari malformation; usually associated with spina bifida
  Posterior fossa arachnoid cyst causing obstruction
  Choroid plexus tumour causing cerebrospinal fluid overproduction
  X-linked hydrocephalus
  Vein of Galen aneurysm
  10% associated with other malfunctions, e.g. trisomy 13, 18, Aicardi syndome

Hydrocephalus acquired in fetal life
  Intracranial haemorrhage due to bleeding disorder
    alloimmune thrombocytopaenia
    factor V or VIII deficiency
    haemorrhage into a tumour or arteriovenous malformation
  In utero infection including toxoplasmosis, cytomegalovirus, varicella

Postnatal hydrocephalus
  Posthaemorrhagic hydrocephalus (birth trauma, GMH-IVH, bleeding
    diathesis)
  Postmeningitic hydrocephalus
  Haemorrhage into a tumour or an arteriovenous malformation
  Obstruction due to an abnormal skull, e.g. Apert's syndrome

Cerebral atrophy

  Cerebral atrophy acquired in fetal life
  Loss of white matter from twin-to-twin transfusion syndrome
  Loss of white matter following maternal collapse, e.g. accident, anaphylaxis

Postnatally acquired cerebral atrophy
  Periventricular white matter damage; causes not yet fully elucidated

be made during fetal life. Table 8.1 summarises the causes of perinatal ventriculomegaly. Ultrasound alone is adequate to confirm the diagnosis in cases of posthaemorrhagic hydrocephalus; Fig. 8.2 shows the typical appearance in a preterm baby, with clot breaking up inside the ventricular cavity (owl's eye) and a ventricular system which is already considerably enlarged. Few neurosurgeons would insist on further imaging before agreeing to operate on this baby if she/he became symptomatic or had a rapid increase in head circumference. Figure 8.3 shows a similar case with massive haemorrhage in the region of the third ventricle causing hydrocephalus. Further investigation, preferably with magnetic resonance imaging, in view of the excellent resolution and the high radiation exposure of CT, is required in less straightforward cases. The resolution in the region of the fourth ventricle is not reliable enough to confirm or refute the diagnosis of aqueduct stenosis. The distinction between very severe congenital hydrocephalus and hydranencephaly is difficult. Viral serology, coagulation

157

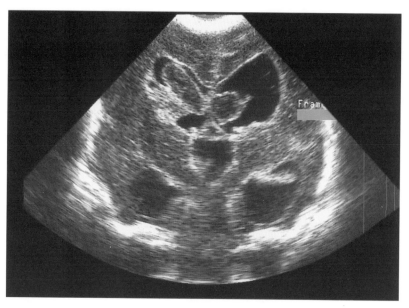

Fig. 8.2. *Posthaemorrhagic hydrocephalus in a preterm child. The ventricles are large and there is an old clot breaking up in both sides.*

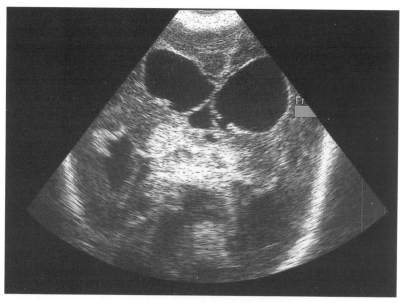

Fig. 8.3. *Posthaemorrhagic hydrocephalus due to a massive area of haemorrhage in the region of the third ventricle and thalamus, appearing bright, and causing an obstructive hydrocephalus.*

studies and maternal platelet typing should be considered if the cause is not obvious (Table 8.1). Haemorrhagic disease of the newborn can cause intracranial bleeding in a term, breast-fed infant. Increased use of oral regimens of vitamin K has already led to a resurgence of this condition (Von Kries *et al.*, 1995), and cerebral haemorrhage due to vitamin K deficiency is often the presenting problem in neonatal cholestasis.

Ultrasound assessment of ventricular size

Linear measurements

The wide range of ventricular size seen in the newborn is shown in Fig. 8.4(a)–(e). In order to define ventriculomegaly for incidence studies, to monitor progress and to minimise inter-observer differences, a reproducible system of measurement is needed. Serial measurements of ventricular size can then be combined with other information, such as serial head circumference and an estimate of the intracranial pressure, to help determine whether surgical intervention is likely to be required. At least six different linear measurement systems have been described (Fig. 8.5) and to these can be added several ratios of ventricle:brain width (Johnson *et al.*, 1979; Garrett *et al.*, 1980; Poland *et al.*, 1985). Zatz (1979), however, casts doubt on the accuracy of these ratios.

London *et al.* (1980) made four linear measurements including the maximum span of the frontal horns, the width of the frontal horn at the level of the caudate nucleus and the intercaudate distance. Allen *et al.* (1982) measured the diameter of the lateral ventricle at the mid-body on a parasagittal scan (E in Fig. 8.5). These authors claimed that this measurement separated cases of progressive from non-progressive hydrocephalus, but did not study any normal infants. Poland *et al.* (1985) carefully studied 67 normal infants but did not evaluate their system in babies with abnormal ventricles. The ventricular index of Levene (1981) was the best documented at the start, with the normal range established from measurements on 273 preterm infants. This index measures the distance from the falx to the lateral border of the lateral ventricle in a coronal view taken in the plane of the third ventricle. The measurement is easy to understand and teach, appears reproducible and has consequently been widely adopted. Ultrasound machines are now fitted with electronic calipers which allow the measurement to be made easily at the cot-side (Fig. 8.6). The large collaborative trial of treatment for ventriculomegaly (Ventriculomegaly Trial Group 1990, 1994) used 4 mm above the 97th centile of Levene to define trial entry, and this proved robust in many different centres. The original centile chart is reproduced as Fig. 8.7 (Levene, 1981). The only disadvantage of Levene's system in clinical practice occurs when there is midline shift, and I have adopted a personal convention of measuring from the midpoint of the ventricular borders rather than the anatomical midline structures in this situation.

159

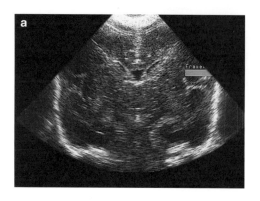

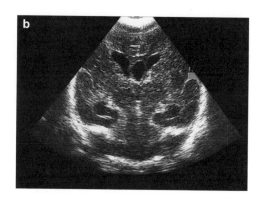

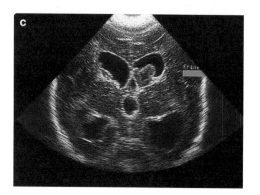

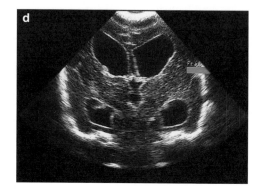

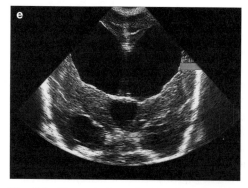

Fig. 8.4. *Coronal views showing the range of ventricular size from normal (a) to massively enlarged (e). The third ventricle is big in (c), (d) and (e).*

160

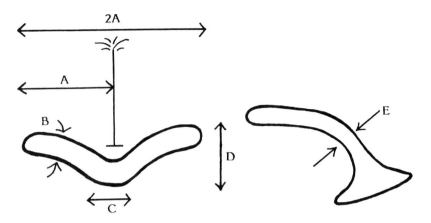

Fig. 8.5. *Different linear measurements which can be made from coronal and para-sagittal scans in ventriculomegaly. (Reproduced with permission of Blackwell, Oxford, from Levene et al., 1985.) A: the ventricular index of Levene (1981), Sauerbrei et al. (1981), Lipscomb et al. (1983); 2A: Skolnick et al. (1979), London et al. (1980); B: London et al. (1980), Sauerbrei et al. (1981); C: London et al. (1980); D: Levene & Starte (1981); E: Allen et al. (1982); Quisling et al. (1983).*

Shackleford (1986) thoroughly reviewed the measurement systems and reinforced the requirement for observers to use a quantitative measurement for the diagnosis of ventriculomegaly, rather than basing a diagnosis on a subjective assessment of the size of the occipital horns. Although the occipital horns do dilate early in ventriculomegaly they are highly variable in size and frequently asymmetrical in normal infants (Shen & Huang, 1989). There are as yet no established ultrasound criteria for diagnosis of enlarged third and fourth ventricles or the cisterna magna in neonates. This last may become pressing as the diagnosis is increasingly suggested in fetal life, and may need postnatal confirmation.

Area measurements

A two-dimensional measurement conveys more information than a one-dimensional measurement. Area calipers are now usually available on commercial ultrasound equipment, allowing the ventricle to be measured in two dimensions with ease. For those without this facility many personal computers can be fitted with a digitising tablet that enable the operator to draw around the irregular shape on a picture (Fig. 8.8), eliminating the laborious step of counting squares on graph paper (Saliba *et al.*, 1990a, b). Tracing the ventricular area with electronic calipers at the cot-side may prolong the time of the investigation but images can be stored for subsequent analysis. The practical difficulties, the additional time taken to measure area and the lack of an easily recognisable landmark with which to standardise the parasagittal view seem to have prevented wide accept-

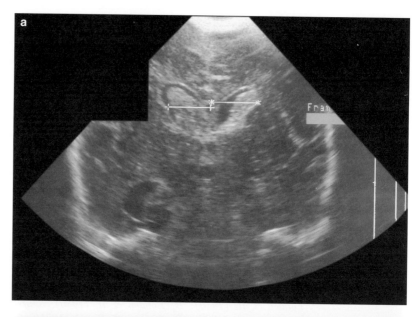

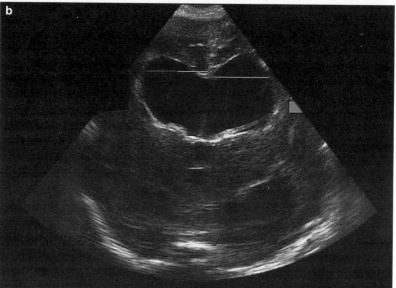

Fig. 8.6. *Coronal scans (a) and (b) showing the Levene ventricular index plotted on the screen using the calipers.*

ance of area measurements. An additional problem is that when the ventricle is very large the boundaries are not always visible in either the parasagittal or coronal plane.

A normal range for area has been defined and used to study outcome (Saliba *et al.*, 1990a, b). The area of the lateral ventricle was measured in a standard coronal plane similar to Fig. 8.6. The area of the ventricular

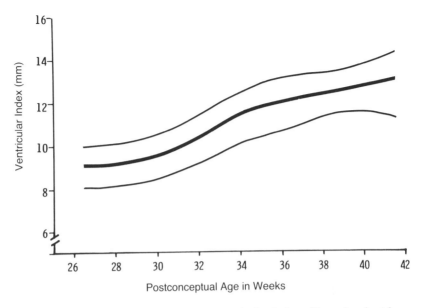

Fig. 8.7. *Centile chart for the Levene ventricular index. (Reproduced with permission from Levene, 1981).*

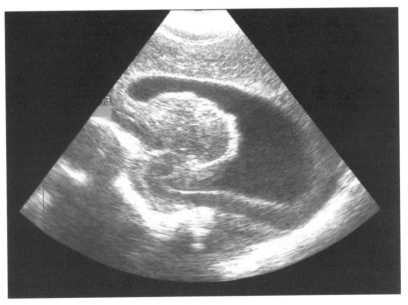

Fig. 8.8. *A parasagittal image of an enlarged ventricle suitble for tracing the area.*

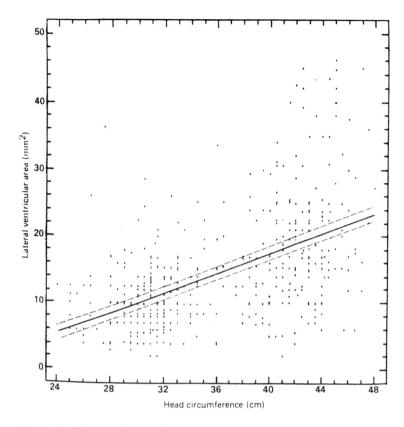

Fig. 8.9. *The normal range for ventricular area related to head circumference (on the X axis). (Reproduced with permission from Saliba et al., 1990b.)*

ellipse ranged from 8 mm^2 to 16 mm^2 (Fig. 8.9), with a growth rate of 0.5 mm^2 per week for the first six weeks after birth. Note that Fig. 8.9 relates area to head circumference not to postconceptional age.

Volume measurements

Undeterred by the lack of enthusiasm for measuring the area of the lateral ventricles, some researchers have quantified ventricular volume. This needs fairly heavy-duty computing power in order to sum the area of serial scans, but the programmes have been adapted from those developed for CT and made to work (Brann *et al.*, 1989a, b). Using volume measurements, the rate of growth was greater (4.2±3.3 ml/day) in those who required intervention than in cases of non-progressive ventriculomegaly (0.0±0.2 ml/day) (Brann *et al.*, 1990). The differences were apparent by the third week of postnatal life. A ventricular volume of more than 30 ml by the seventeenth day gave a 90% chance that the ventriculomegaly would progress. Using the same method, this group have shown a third order polynomial relationship between the ventricular index and volume and

164

confirmed beyond doubt the observation that the occipital horn enlarges most rapidly in hydrocephalus (Brann *et al.*, 1991).

Doppler ultrasound studies of ventriculomegaly

The hope that Doppler ultrasound measurement of cerebral blood flow velocity would be able to provide a non-invasive estimate of intracranial pressure has not so far been realised. The studies are summarised in Table 5.3; all report a change in the ratio of systolic:diastolic velocity with most observing an increase in systolic velocity and a reduction in diastolic velocity leading to an increase in the Pourcelot index which relates the two. There are insufficient data to base a clinical decision on Doppler ultrasound results at present.

Monitoring ventriculomegaly

Distinguishing progressive from non-progressive ventriculomegaly

Once enlarged cerebral ventricles have been diagnosed it is essential to plot all previously available head circumference measurements on a suitable centile chart. A lumbar puncture or ventricular tap should be done to measure intracranial pressure, and to examine cerebrospinal fluid. This may be the only way of detecting low-grade ventriculitis that may have no other manifestations (Waites *et al.*, 1988). Ultrasound can be used to guide a ventricular tap if lumbar puncture is difficult (Levene, 1982). The combination of rapidly enlarging ventricles and high intracranial pressure (15 cm of cerebrospinal fluid in a preterm baby) with symptoms of lethargy, apnoea or convulsions would be an indication for considering early surgical intervention. Insertion of a ventricular catheter with a reservoir can be done on the neonatal unit in infants too small or sick to tolerate placement of a ventriculoperitoneal shunt. In infants with more slowly enlarging ventricles a decision to intervene is based on the head circumference crossing centile lines and/or the presence of symptoms and signs of raised intracranial pressure. Progression is more likely if the cerebrospinal fluid pressure is above 10 cm but at present early prediction of later shunt dependence is impossible. Frequent intermittent aspiration of cerebrospinal fluid in this situation cannot prevent progression and infection is a risk (Ventriculomegaly Trial Group, 1990). Other forms of management including acetazolamide and frusemide, or intraventricular fibrinolysis, are undergoing evaluation. Babies whose ventriculomegaly resolves in the neonatal period require monitoring for up to a year, as late hydrocephalus can develop (Perlman *et al.*, 1990).

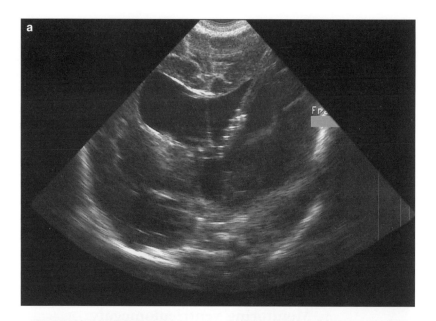

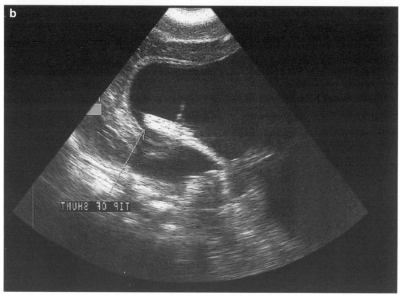

Fig. 8.10. *Appearance of a well-placed ventricular catheter, (a) coronal and (b) parasagittal views.*

Checking the position of intraventricular catheters

Fortunately intraventricular catheters are highly echogenic and easy to see with ultrasound. The catheter in Fig. 8.10 is in a good position with the tip anterior, well away from the choroid plexus which can obstruct the holes. The ventricular part of the catheter is deep within the ventricle

166

and surrounded by cerebrospinal fluid. Occasionally clot forms around the catheter postoperatively, and this can be identified with ultrasound. Ultrasound can also assess the rate of reduction of ventricular size after surgery. Over-drainage can produce a slit ventricle syndrome in later childhood resulting from loss of compliance of the ventricular walls which cannot re-expand to accomodate increased cerebrospinal fluid. Children with this syndrome rapidly become symptomatic if the shunt blocks. Ventricles which are not in free communication due to adhesions drain asymmetrically, a 'trapped ventricle'. Ultrasound has been used to identify loculated collections of cerebrospinal fluid in the peritoneal cavity in cases of shunt malfunction (Briggs *et al.*, 1984), although an X-ray is required to diagnose disconnection. Recently colour Doppler ultrasound has been used to demonstrate a flash from flow of cerebrospinal fluid in the subcutaneous catheter.

References

Allen, W.C., Holt, P.J., Sawyer, I.R., Tito, A.M. & Meade, S.K. (1982) Ventricular dilatation after neonatal periventricular-intraventricular haemorrhage. *American Journal of Diseases of Children*, **136**:589–93.

Brann, B.S., Wofsy, C., Papile, L.A., Angelus, P. & Backstrom, C. (1989a) The quantification of neonatal cerebral ventricular volume by real time ultrasonography: *in vivo* validation of the cylindrical co-ordinate method. *Journal of Ultrasound in Medicine*, **9**:9–15.

Brann, B.S., Wofsy, C., Wicks, J. & Brayer, J. (1989b) The quantification of neonatal cerebral ventricular volume by real time ultrasonography: derivation and *in vitro* comfirmation of a mathematical model. *Journal of Ultrasound in Medicine*, **9**:1–8.

Brann, B.S., Qualls, C., Papile, L.A., Wells, L. & Werner, S. (1990) Measurement of progressive cerebral ventriculomegaly in infants after grades III and IV intraventricular haemorrhage. *Journal of Pediatrics*, **117**:615–21.

Brann, B.S., Qualls, C., Wells, L. & Papile, L.A. (1991) Asymmetric growth of the lateral cerebral ventricle in infants with posthemorrhagic ventricular dilatation. *Journal of Pediatrics*, **118**:108–12.

Briggs , J.R., Hendry, G.M.A. & Minns, R.A. (1984) Abdominal ultrasound in the diagnosis of cerebrospinal fluid pseudocysts complicating ventriculoperitoneal shunts. *Archives of Disease in Childhood*, **59**:661–4.

Garrett, W.J., Kossoff, G. & Warren, P.A. (1980) Cerebral ventricular size in children: a two dimensional ultrasonographic study. *Radiology*, **136**:711–15.

Hill, A. & Volpe, J.J. (1981) Normal pressure hydrocephalus in the newborn. *Pediatrics*, **68**:623–9.

Kaiser, A. & Whitelaw, A. (1985) Cerebrospinal fluid pressure during posthaemorrhagic ventriculomegaly in newborn infants. *Archives of Disease in Childhood*, **60**:920–4.

Johnson, M.L., Mack, L.A., Rumack, C.M., Frost, M. & Rashbaum, C.L. (1979) B mode echoencephalography in the normal and high risk infant. *American Journal of Radiology*, **133**:375–81.

Levene, M.I. (1981) Measurement of the growth of the lateral ventricles in preterm infants with real time ultrasound. *Archives of Disease in Childhood*, **56**:900–4.

Levene, M.I. (1982) Ventricular tap under direct ultrasound control. *Archives of Disease in Childhood*, **57**:873–4.

Levene, M.I. & Starte, D.R. (1981) A longitudinal study of post-haemorrhagic ventricular dilatation in the newborn. *Archives of Disease in Childhood*, **58**:905–10.

Levene, M.I., Williams, J.L. & Fawer, C.-L. (1985) *Ultrasound of the Infant Brain. Clinics in Developmental Medicine*, No 92. Spastics International Medical Publications. Oxford: Blackwell.

Lipscomb, A.P., Thorburn, R.J., Stewart, A.L., Reynolds, E.O.R. & Hope, P.L. (1983) Early treatment for rapidly progressive ventricular dilatation in the newborn. *Lancet*, **i**:1438–9.

London, D.A., Carroll, B.A. & Enzmann, D.R. (1980) Sonography of ventricular size and germinal matrix hemorrhage in premature infants. *American Journal of Neuroradiolology*, **1**:295–300.

Perlman, J.M., Lynch, B. & Volpe, J.J. (1990) Late hydrocephalus after arrest and resolution of neonatal posthaemorrhagic hydrocephalus. *Developmental Medicine and Child Neurology*, **32**:725–42.

Poland, R.L., Slovis, T.L. & Shankaran, S. (1985) Normal values for ventricular size as determined by real time ultrasonography. *Pediatric Radiology*, **15**:12–14.

Quisling, R.G., Reeder, J.D., Setzer, E.S. & Kaude, J.V. (1983) Ultrasonic evaluation of neonatal intracranial haemorrhage and its complications. *Neuroradiology*, **24**:205–11.

Saliba, E., Bertrand, P., Gold, F., Marchand. S. & Laugier, J. (1990a) Area of lateral ventricles measured on cranial ultrasonography in preterm infants: association with outcome. *Archives of Disease in Childhood*, **65**:1035–7.

Saliba, E., Bertrand, P., Gold, F., Valliant, M.C. & Laugier, J. (1990b) Area of lateral ventricles measured on cranial ultrasonography in preterm infants: reference range. *Archives of Disease in Childhood*, **65**:1029–32.

Sauerbrei, E.E., Digney, M., Harrison, P.B. & Cooperberg, P.L. (1981) Ultrasonic evaluation of neonatal intracranial haemorrhage and its complications. *Radiology*, **139**:677–85.

Shackleford, G.D. (1986) Neurosonography of hydrocephalus in infants. *Neuroradiology*, **28**:452–62.

Shen, E-Y. & Huang, F-Y. (1989) Sonographic finding of ventricular asymmetry in neonatal brain. *Archives of Disease in Childhood*, **64**:730–44.

Skolnick, M.L., Rosenbaum, A.E., Matzuk, T., Guthkelch, A.N. & Heinz, E.R. (1979) Detection of dilated cerebral ventricles in infants: a correlative study between ultrasound and computed tomography. *Radiology*, **131**:447–52.

Ventriculomegaly Trial Group (1990) Randomised trial of early tapping in neonatal posthaemorrhagic ventricular dilatation. *Archives of Disease in Childhood*, **65**:3–10.

Ventriculomegaly Trial Group (1994) Randomised trial of early tapping in neonatal posthaemorrhagic ventricular dilatation: results at 30 months. *Archives of Disease in Childhood*, **70**:F129–F136.

Von Kries, R., Hachmeister, A. & Göbel, U. (1995) Repeated oral vitamin K prophylaxis in West Germany: acceptance and efficacy. *British Medical Journal*, **310**:1097–8.

Waites, K.B., Rudd, P.T., Crouse, D.T., Canupp, K.C., Nelson, K.G., Ramsey, C. & Cassell, G.H. (1988) Chronic ureaplasma, urealyticum and mycoplasma hominis infections of the central nervous system in preterm infants. *Lancet* i:17–21.

Zatz, L.M. (1979) The Evans ratio for ventricular size: a calculation error. *Neuro-radiology*, **18**:81.

9 *Infection*

Introduction

Ultrasound can contribute to diagnosis and management of central nervous system infection. As with hypoxic-ischaemic encephalopathy, ventriculomegaly and germinal matrix haemorrhage-intraventricular haemorrhage (GMH-IVH), the main strength of ultrasound is the ability to image a sick infant repeatedly without undue disturbance.

Congenital infection

Cytomegalovirus

Multiple periventricular cysts, intraventricular strands, ventriculomegaly and intracranial calcification have all been described in cases of congenital cytomegalovirus (CMV) infection (Dykes *et al.*, 1982; Butt *et al.*, 1984; Fawer, 1985; Teele *et al.*, 1988; Toma *et al.*, 1989; Ben-Ami *et al.*, 1990; Weber *et al.*, 1992). Figure 9.1 shows extensive areas of pinpoint calcification in a term infant who presented with classical CMV; he had jaundice, petechiae and hepatosplenomegaly – a 'bluberry muffin' baby. Figure 9.2 shows lace like cystic change in the subependymal region. This infant was small for dates at term and was proven to have congenital CMV infection; at two years of age she was found to be normal. Weber *et al.* (1992) describe finding hyperechoic lesions in the basal ganglia in 15 (0.4%) of 3600 screened newborns. CMV infection was proven in only two, and in most of the remaining children no cause was found. Other possible explanations for calcification in the thalamic region include infections such as congenital rubella syndrome (Carey *et al.*, 1987) and AIDS (Epstein *et al.*, 1987). Hypoxic-ischaemic encephalopathy (see Chapter 11) and meningitis can also cause thalamic calcification but in some children it appears to be an incidental finding.

Toxoplasmosis, rubella

Both these intrauterine infections can cause intracranial lesions similar to those occurring in CMV infection with calcification and cyst formation. In addition toxoplasmosis in the first trimester can cause malformations such as hydranencephaly.

170

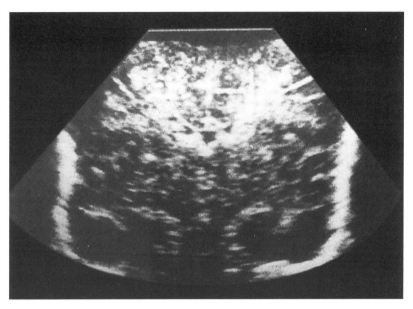

Fig. 9.1. *Coronal scan showing extensive periventricular calcification in a case of congenital cytomegalovirus infection.*

Meningitis

All cases of neonatal meningitis should be monitored with cranial ultrasound to detect dilatation of the cerebral ventricles. Ventriculomegaly occurs in as many as 60% of cases (Edwards *et al.*, 1982; Perlman *et al.*, 1992). Strands can be seen in the ventricular cavity in ventriculitis, probably due to inflammatory exudate (Hill *et al.*, 1981; Reeder & Sanders, 1983). The strands look like a cobweb within the ventricle (Fig. 9.3). Purulent exudate sometimes forms debris which accumulates within the ventricle, settling out with gravity but remaining mobile. When the infant's head is moved during an ultrasound examination the particles whirl about like the particles in a toy paperweight snow scene. These sonographic signs, particularly in a case where the patient is not responding to treatment, are an indication for a ventricular tap and consideration of intraventricular therapy (Rennie, 1995). Intraventricular septum formation can wall off part of the ventricular system which then later fails to drain adequately – the 'trapped ventricle' syndrome.

Periventricular echodensity has also been described in neonatal meningitis, particularly with virulent organisms such as *Proteus* (Rosenberg *et al.*, 1983). These areas can form abscess cavities – citrobacter has a predilection for abcess formation in the newborn (Kline 1988). Thalamic echodensities have been mentioned as a possible indicator of congenital infection or hypoxic-ischaemic encephalopathy but have also been desribed in meningitis. Figure 9.4 shows a bright spot of thalamic calcification in a

171

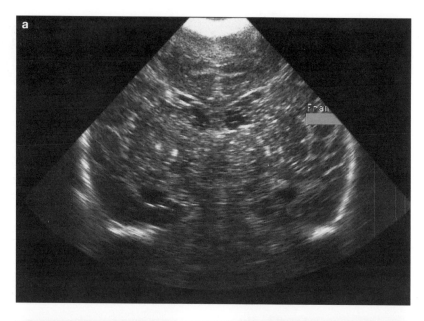

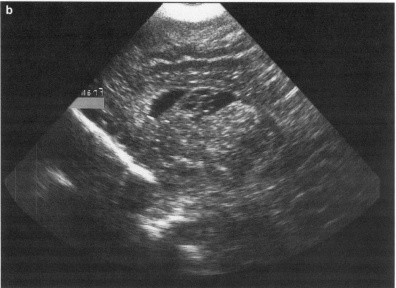

Fig. 9.2. *Coronal (a) and parasagittal (b) scans showing subependymal cystic change in a case of congenital cytomegalovirus infection.*

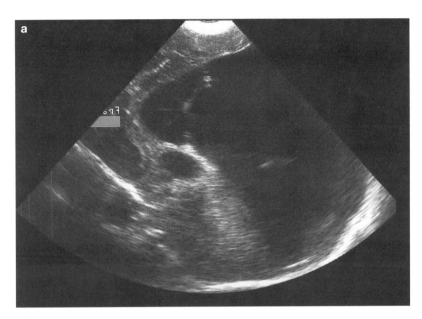

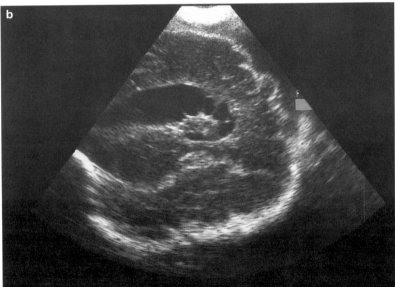

Fig. 9.3. *Parsagittal scans in a case of neonatal ventriculitis, showing a cobweb appearance of strands of fibrin.*

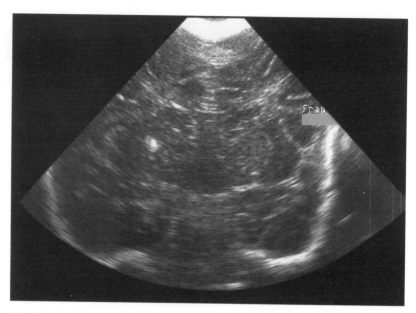

Fig. 9.4. *Parasagittal scan showing a bright spot of calcification in the thalamic region in a case of* Escherichia coli *neonatal meningitis.*

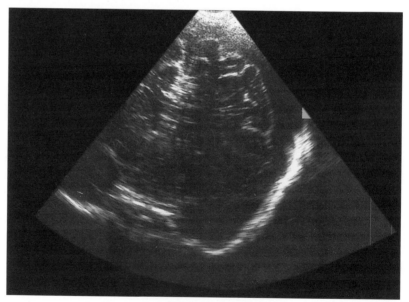

Fig. 9.5. *Subdural effusion in pneumococcal meningitis.*

neonate suffering from *Escherichia coli* meningitis. He was discharged from the clinic at two years of age when he was entirely normal. Similar lesions have been reported by others and were thought to represent vasculitis or a small venous infarction (Perlman *et al.*, 1992; Weber *et al.*, 1992).

Subdural effusions are not well seen with ultrasound unless they are large (Fig. 9.5). CT or magnetic resonance imaging (MRI) scanning may be required if there is a high index of suspicion but need not be routine in neonatal meningitis.

References

Ben-Ami, T., Yousefzadeh, D., Backus, M., Reichman, B., Kessler, A. & Hammerman-Rozenberg, C. (1990) Lenticulostriate vasculopathy in infants with infections of the central nervous system: sonographic and Doppler findings. *Pediatric Radiology*, **20**:575–9.

Butt, W., Mackay, R.J., De Crespigny, L., Murton, L.J. & Roy, R.N.D. (1984) Intracranial lesions of congenital cytomegalovirus infection detected by ultrasound scanning. *Pediatrics*, **73**:611–14.

Carey, B.M., Arthur, R.J. & Houlsby, W.T. (1987) Ventriculitis in congenital rubella: Ultrasound demonstration. *Pediatric Radiology*, **17**:415–16.

Dykes, F.D., Ahmann, P.A. & Lazzara, A. (1982) Cranial ultrasound in the detection of intracranial calcification. *Journal of Pediatrics*, **100**:406–8.

Edwards, M.K., Brown, D.L. & Chua, G.T. (1982) Complicated infantile meningitis: Evaluation by real-time sonography. *American Journal of Neuroradiology*, **3**:431–4.

Epstein, L.G., Berman, C.Z., Sharer, L.R., Khademi, M. & Desposito, F. (1987) Unilateral calcification and contrast enhancement of the basal ganglia in a child with AIDS encephalopathy. *American Journal of Neuroradiology*, **8**:163–5.

Fawer, C.-L. (1985) Infection. In *Ultrasound of the Infant Brain*, ed. M.I. Levene, J.L. Williams & C.-L. Fawer, pp. 110–17. *Clinics in Developmental Medicine* No. 92. London: Spastics International Medical Publications.

Hill, A., Shackleford, G.D. & Volpe, J.J. (1981) Ventriculitis with neonatal meningitis: identification with real-time ultrasound. *Journal of Pediatrics*, **99**:133–6.

Kline, M.W. (1988) Citrobacter meningitis and brain abscess in infancy: epidemiology, pathogenesis and treatment. *Journal of Pediatrics*, **113**:430–4.

Perlman, J.M., Rollins, N. & Sanchez, P.J. (1992) Late onset meningitis in sick, very low birthweight infants. *American Journal of Diseases in Children*, **146**:1297–301.

Reeder, J.D. & Sanders, R.C. (1983) Ventriculitis in the neonate: recognition by sonography. *American Journal of Neuroradiology*, **4**:37–41.

Rennie, J.M. (1995) Bacterial and fungal infections. In *Fetal and Neonatal Neurology and Neurosurgery*, ed. M.I. Levene & R.J. Lilford, pp. 473–99. Edinburgh: Churchill Livingstone.

Rosenberg, H.K., Levine, R.S. & Smith, D.R. (1983) Bacerial meningitis in infants: sonographic features. *American Journal of Neuroradiology*, **4**:822–5.

Teele, R.L., Hernanz-Schulman, M. & Sotrel, A. (1988) Echogenic vasculature in the basal ganglia of neonates: a sonographic sign of vasculopathy. *Radiology*, **169**: 423–7.

Toma, P., Magnano, G.M., Mezzano, P., Lazzinni, F., Bonacci, W. & Serra,

G. (1989) Cerebral ultrasound images in prenatal cytomegalovirus infection. *Neuroradiology*, 31:278–9.

Weber, K., Riebel, Th. & Nasir, R. (1992) Hyperechoic lesions in the basal ganglia: an incidental sonographic finding in neonates and infants. *Pediatric Radiology*, 22:182–6.

10 *Congential malformations*

Introduction

A discussion of the vast range of complex congenital malformations of the brain is beyond the scope of this book, so I will discuss only those conditions that can be diagnosed using ultrasound. Often the full range of imaging techniques will be required, particularly if neurosurgery is a possibility. Ultrasound can be a helpful first step and should be used to look for a midline defect in babies with a cleft palate or hypertelorism. Sometimes ultrasound gives a better impression of the character of the defect than MRI or CT; for example, we have found this in some arachnoid cysts.

Disorders of prosencephalic development

Holoprosencephaly

In its most severe form (alobar holoprosencephaly) there is a single-sphered cerebral structure with a common ventricle, absent olefactory bulbs and optic tracts, and the facial anomaly (Fig. 10.1) gives the clue to the underlying problem. There may be a single median eye or severe hypotelorism, a single-nostril nose (cebocephaly) with or without a proboscis and/or a cleft lip and palate. Cranial ultrasound reveals the single ventricle straddling fused thalami (Fig. 10.2). Similar pathology is shown in Fig. 10.3. Holoprosencephaly can be a feature of trisomy 13 or 15. Careful examination of the parents is important as there is a rare dominant form in which the carrier can have subtle midline defects such as a single maxillary incisor tooth (Berry *et al.*, 1984).

Agenesis of the septum pellucidum

The septum pellucidum can be destroyed by hydrocephalus, or its absence can be associated with malformations of the brain such as septo-optic dysplasia. The full syndrome of septo-optic dysplasia includes absence of the septum pellucidum, optic nerve hypoplasia, absence or thinning of the corpus callosum and hypothalamic-pituitary dysfunction. Because of the associated midline defects of the face and brain this anomaly has been regarded as part of the spectrum including holoprosencephaly and agenesis

177

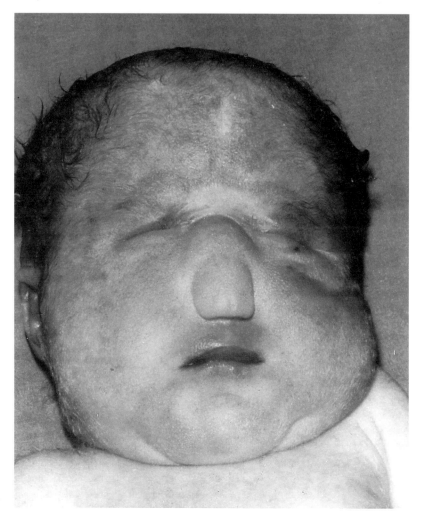

Fig. 10.1. *Facial anomaly in holoprosencephaly.*

of the corpus callosum (Leech & Shuman, 1986). Mildly affected children have visual deficit but no intellectual impairment, implying that in many reports where the children were retarded the cause was due to the associated cerebral hemisphere malformations rather than loss of the septum pellucidum alone (Williams *et al.*, 1993). The falx is present in septo-optic dysplasia and usually absent in holoprosencephaly. Ultrasound diagnosis, both in prenatal and postnatal life, has been described (Pilu *et al.*, 1990).

Occasionally the two leaves of the septum pellucidum may fail to fuse; this is normal in preterm infants who have a large cavum septum pellucidum. However, if this structure is more than 1 cm wide in term infants further investigation is indicated; in one series of nine children, eight had

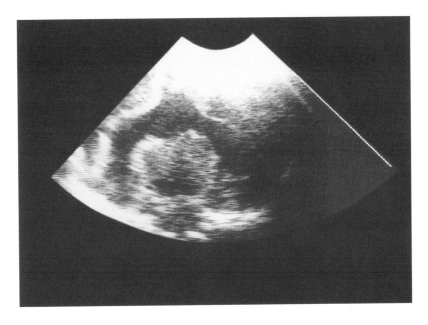

Fig. 10.2. *Ultrasound scan in the baby shown in Fig. 10.1; there is a common horseshoe-shaped ventricle and fused thalami.*

cognitive impairments and four had hypothalamic disturbances (Boden-steiner & Shaefer, 1990).

Agenesis of the corpus callosum

Agenesis of the corpus callosum can be an isolated abnormality, in which case there is usually no detectable neurological abnormality unless sophisticated tests of interhemispheric processing are used. The importance, like that of an absent septum pellucidum, lies in the association with other abnormalities. Aicardi's syndrome occurs in females and consists of partial or complete agenesis of the corpus callosum, infantile spasms and chorio-retinal lacunae. The condition can also be associated with disorders of neuronal migration or trisomy 8. The ultrasound appearances are characteristic and the diagnosis can be made in fetal life (Sandri *et al.*, 1988). The normal corpus callosum is usually easily visualised in the midline, with the pericallosal sulcus forming a clear 'tram-line' band in the midline sagittal and coronal views (Babcock, 1984). In the absence of the corpus callosum the third ventricle often appears high and between the lateral ventricles (this can vary), which are widely separated and of abnormal shape. They appear like butterfly wings on the coronal scan (Fig. 10.4), with a flat lateral border (Sheehy-Skeffington, 1982). There is loss of the normal convexity of the medial borders of the anterior horns of the lateral ventricles (Hernanz-Schulman *et al.*, 1985). In the parasagittal view the

179

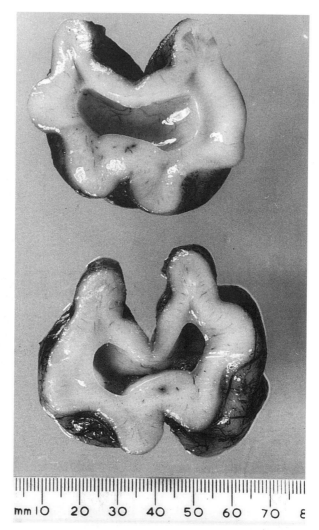

Fig. 10.3. *Pathological specimen of an infant with holoprosencephaly.*

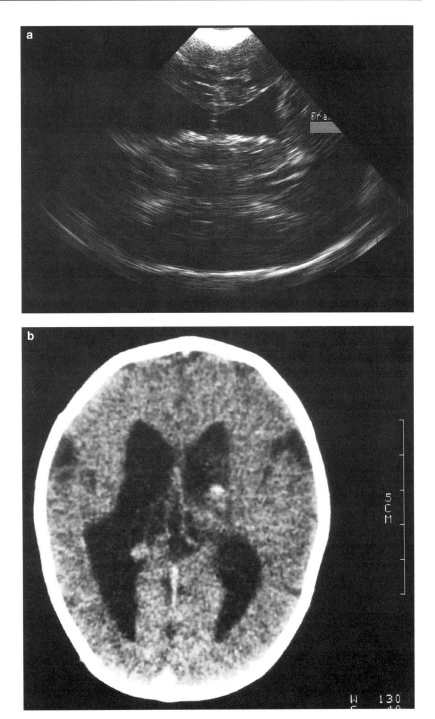

Fig. 10.4. *Coronal scan (a) and computed tomography scan (b) showing agenesis of the corpus callosum.*

cortical sulci radiate superiorly instead of horizontally, giving rise to a sunburst appearance (Volpe, 1995).

Agenesis of the cerebellum

Hypoplasia of the cerebellum occurs more often than complete agenesis, and can be diagnosed with ultrasound although the posterior fossa is difficult to image. Agenesis of the cerebellar vermis can be associated with the Dandy-Walker malformation or can occur as part of Joubert's syndrome. In this familial disorder, infants present with effortless panting tachypnoea and rhythmic tongue and eye movements; the children are retarded (Joubert *et al.*, 1969).

Disorders of neural tube development

Arnold-Chiari malformation

Nearly every case of thoracolumbar, lumbar or lumbosacral myelomeningocoele is accompanied by the Arnold-Chiari malformation which is central to the development of hydrocephalus. The cerebellum is displaced downwards into the foramen magnum. There are bony deficits of the foramen magnum and upper cervical vertebrae. The fourth ventricle and the medulla are displaced into the upper cervical canal. There is aqueduct stenosis in 40–75% of cases. The severe hydrocephalus associated with an Arnold-Chiari malformation is shown in Fig. 10.5; there is loss of the septum pellucidum which is typical of longstanding prenatal hydrocephalus. Figure 10.6 shows the midline sagittal appearances of the Arnold-Chiari malformation; the fourth ventricle is low.

Disorders of neuronal proliferation

Schizencephaly

In this very severe disorder there appears to be a complete agenesis of a portion of germinal matrix so that a whole area of brain fails to develop, leaving a seam or cleft in the cerebral hemisphere. The lips of the clefts can become widely separated, and they tend to be in the area of the Rolandic or Sylvian fissure. The advent of MRI has revealed that this condition is not as rare as was thought, and ultrasound has been used to diagnose the abnormality (Pellicer *et al.*, 1995).

Lissencephaly

Lissencephaly means 'smooth brain' and is believed to result from a complete interruption of neuronal migration from the germinal matrix to the brain surface. The brain has no or very few gyri. When the disorder occurs

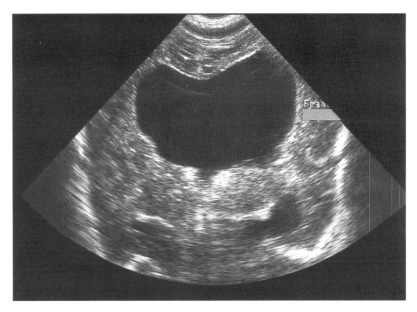

Fig. 10.5. *Hydrocephalus associated with the Arnold–Chiari malformation. There is agenesis of the septum pellucidum.*

in conjunction with other malformations such as cardiac defects, genital abnormalities, characteristic facies including a long upper lip with a tip-tilted nose, the Miller-Dieker syndrome may be present. In many cases there is a deletion of part of the short arm of chromosome 17, which can be a micro-deletion. In some cases a ring chromosome 17 has been observed. Lissencephaly can be visualised with ultrasound (Babcock, 1983) and features include a lack of the Y shape of the Sylvian fissure on coronal views and there is no operculisation of the insula. Confirmation of ultrasound diagnosis with CT or MRI is desirable, but several authors have successfully imaged neuronal migration disorders (Trounce *et al.*, 1986; Pellicer *et al.*, 1995).

Congenital cystic disorders

Hydranencephaly

The whole of both hemispheres is missing in this condition, thought to arise from an *in utero* occlusion of both carotid arteries or a massive hypotensive insult to the fetus (maternal collapse or death of a co-twin). There is a residual thin mantle of meninges and the skull is normally formed. The structures which are supplied by the posterior cerebral circulation remain intact, namely the brain stem, the occipital lobes and the basal ganglia (Fig. 10.7). The falx is preserved. EEG is sometimes helpful in distinguishing hydranencephaly from severe hydrocephalus (Sutton *et al.*,

183

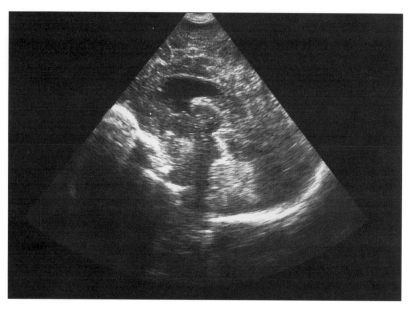

Fig. 10.6. *Sagittal image of the Arnold–Chiari malformation in an infant with spina bifida.*

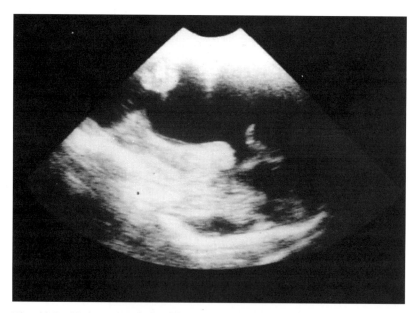

Fig. 10.7. *Hydrancencephaly. The cortex is filled with fluid. The basal ganglia and the brainstem are intact.*

1980). Management is similar in that an expanding head circumference is an indication for insertion of a ventriculoperitoneal shunt.

Dandy-Walker cysts

The term Dandy-Walker cyst is used to refer to cystic lesions in the posterior fossa. A true Dandy-Walker malformation results from atresia of the foramen of Magendie and Lushka, with partial agenesis of the cerebellar vermis resulting in massive dilation of the fourth ventricle. The Dandy-Walker variant has an identical appearance with the addition of a communication into the perimedullary spaces through the foramen of Magendie which is patent. Arachnoid cysts in this region and cysts of the cisterna magna can cause confusion but in these conditions the fourth ventricle is of normal size. Figure 10.8 (a)–(c) shows the ultrasound appearances of a Dandy-Walker cyst expanding the posterior fossa; Fig. 10.9 show the CT scans from the same case.

Arachnoid cysts

Arachnoid cysts contain cerebrospinal fluid which is secreted from their lining. They cause symptoms when they expand and displace normal brain. Arachnoid cysts can occur in conjunction with hydrocephalus; Fig. 10.10 shows a cyst present as the underlying cause in a case of hydrocephalus. Ultrasound (Fig. 10.11a,b) sometimes gives a better impression than CT (Fig. 10.11c) of the anatomy within these cysts.

Choroid plexus cysts

Choroid plexus cysts are seen in about 1% of prenatal scans of the fetal brain. They were initially thought to be a marker of chromosomal abnormality but it is now thought that they are of no prognostic significance, especially if an isolated finding. Fetal choroid plexus cysts usually disappear by term, but persistence into neonatal life has been described (Lodeiro *et al.*, 1989; Riebel *et al.*, 1992). Persistence does not carry any additional prognostic importance although most continue unchanged (Fig. 10.12). Lam & Villanueva (1992) described three infants in whom the cysts were situated at the foramen of Munro and caused obstructive hydrocephalus. Symptomatic cysts tend to be larger than normal (>2 cm) (Fakhry *et al.*, 1985). Standard CT and MRI failed to reveal the lesions which were correctly identified with ultrasound. Choroid plexus cysts should be distinguished from subependymal cysts by their location well within the body of the choroid plexus.

Leptomeningeal cyst

This lesion is better termed 'growing skull fracture' and is discussed in Chapter 7.

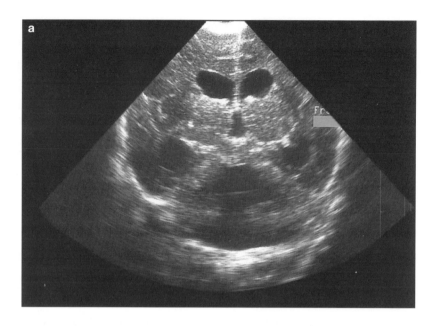

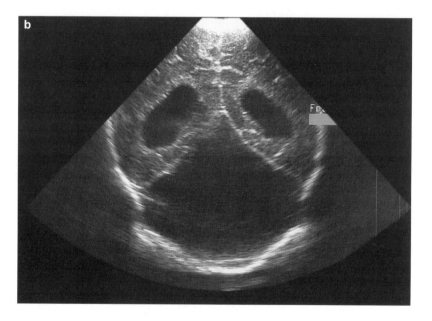

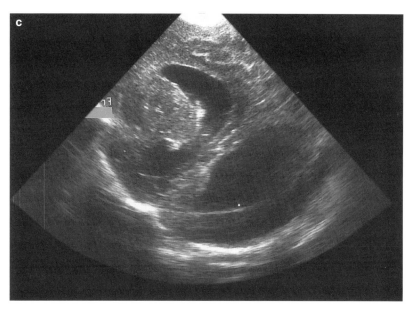

Fig. 10.8. *Coronal scan (a) of Dandy–Walker cyst. The fourth ventricle is replaced by a fluid-filled area, which expands the posterior fossa, seen in (b) which is an occipital coronal scan. The parasagittal view is shown in (c).*

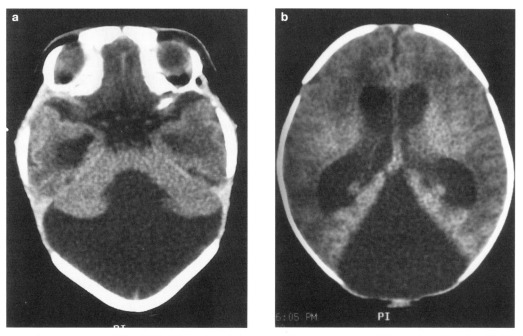

Fig. 10.9. *Two computed tomography scans (a) and (b) showing a Dandy–Walker cyst.*

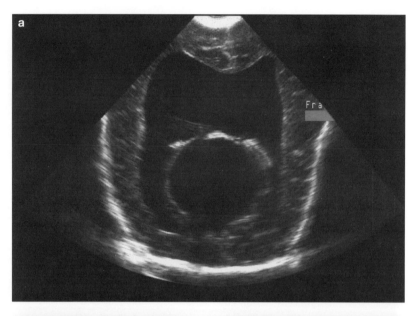

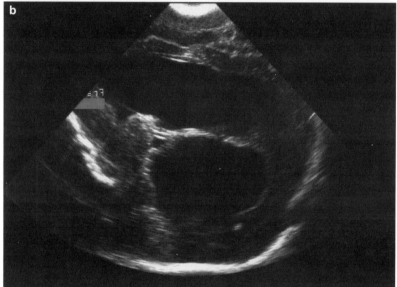

Fig. 10.10. *Ultrasound scans in coronal (a) and parasagittal (b) planes showing a large arachnoid cyst and hydrocephalus.*

Subependymal pseudocysts

With the advent of routine cranial ultrasonography cystic lesions present at the time of delivery have been recognised both in the subependymal region and at the external angle of the lateral ventricle in between 2% and 5% of subjects (Levene, 1980; Shen & Huang, 1985; Keller *et al.*, 1987; Zorzi & Angonese, 1989; Rademaker *et al.*, 1993). The cysts appear like strings of beads along the floor of the lateral ventricle almost septating it (Fig. 10.13). The diagnosis is important as these cysts must be distinguished from periventricular leukomalacia or the sequelae of germinal matrix haemorrhage. The term pseudocyst arises from the pathological description of cysts present at birth, situated in the remnants of the geminal zone at the external angle of the lateral ventricle which were lined with immature cells (Larroche, 1972). The ultrasound appearances correspond to the pathological description. Subependymal pseudocysts have an excellent prognosis; all but one of the 24 survivors followed for a year were normal (Rademaker *et al.*, 1993). Lu *et al.* (1992) found similar cysts in 12 cases during a five-year period of ultrasound screening in Bonn, Germany; they found evidence of congenital viral infection in three and a chromosomal abnormality in one. The illustrations in some cases appear identical to that of Fig. 10.13 and those of Rademaker *et al.* (1993) and it appears that the babies with viral infection had more extensive lesions.

Congenital tumours

Discovery of a brain tumour in the neonatal period is very rare indeed (Sauerbrei & Cooperberg, 1983). They are more likely to come to light if they cause hydrocephalus, and lipomas of the corpus callosum and choroid plexus papillomas have been described (Chuang & Harwood-Nash, 1986; Auriemma *et al.*, 1993).

Congenital vascular lesions

Aneurysm of the vein of Galen

This is an important diagnosis to make as treatment can be life-saving. Infants usually present with intractable heart failure and are sometimes cyanosed. Consequently attention is focused on excluding a cardiac cause and cranial auscultation is forgotten. The sonographic appearances are well described (Sauerbrei & Cooperberg, 1981; Cubberley *et al.*, 1982; Jones *et al.*, 1982). The aneurysm appears as a large cystic structure in the region of the third ventricle. The vascular nature of the space can be elegantly confirmed with colour Doppler which reveals blood flow within the structure; if colour Doppler imaging is not available the older technique of bubble echo can be used – microbubbles present within any injected fluid can obscure the cavity for several seconds after an intravenous injection

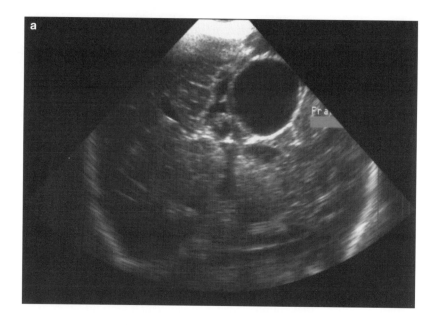

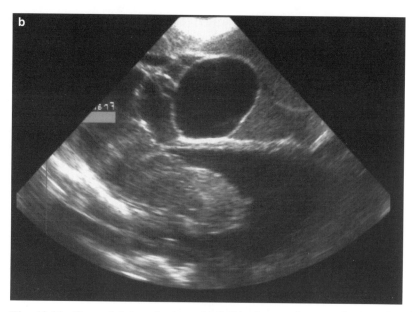

Fig. 10.11. *Coronal (a) and parasagittal (b) ultrasound scans of subarachnoid cyst; shown in computed tomography scan in (c).*

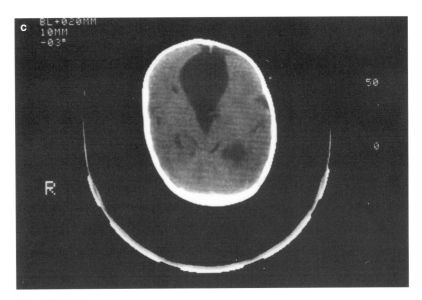

Fig. 10.11 (c).

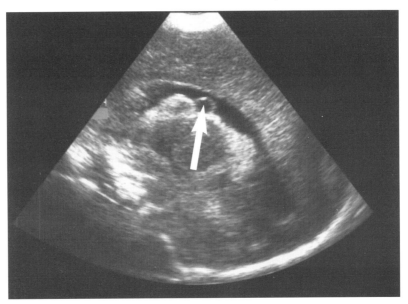

Fig. 10.12. *Persisting choroid plexus cyst (arrowed) from fetal life, in a neonate.*

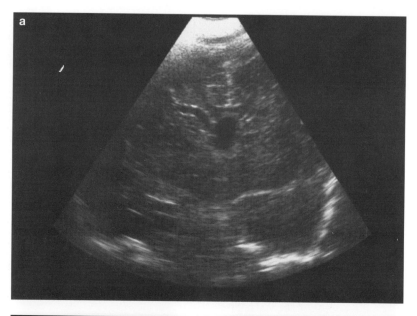

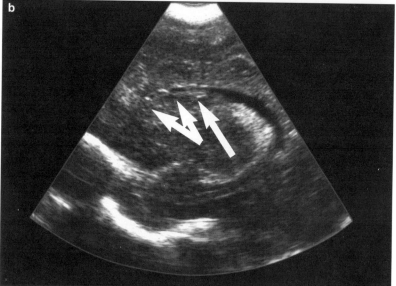

Fig. 10.13. *Subependymal pseudocysts seen in coronal (a) and parasagittal (b, arrowed) scans.*

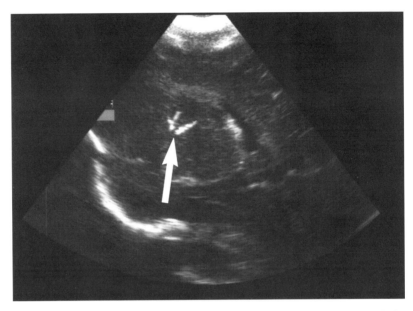

Fig. 10.14. *Vascular calcification in the thalamus seen on a parasagittal ultrasound scan.*

(Tessler *et al.*, 1989; Vaksmann *et al.*, 1989; Deeg & Scharf, 1990; Sirry *et al.*, 1995). Previously the mortality was 100% but since the introduction of embolisation, 30–45% may survive with a good outcome (Lylyk *et al.*, 1993).

Vascular calcification

Bright thalamic vessels have been recognised within the spectrum of thalamic lesions discussed in Chapter 9. Vascular calcification as seen in Fig. 10.14 can indicate congenital cytomegalovirus infection (Teele *et al.*, 1988), although in this case the only possible predisposing factor was abnormal uterine vessel flow demonstrated by antenatal Doppler studies.

References

Auriemma, A., Poggiani, C., Menghini, P., Bellan, C. & Colombo, A. (1993) Lipoma of the corpus callosum in a neonate: sonographic evaluation. *Pediatric Radiology*, **23**:155–6.

Babcock, D.S. (1983) Sonographic demonstration of lissencephaly (Agyria). *Journal of Ultrasound in Medicine*, **2**:465–6.

Babcock, D.S. (1984) The normal, absent and abnormal corpus callosum: sonographic findings. *Radiology*, **151**:449–53.

Berry, S.A., Pierpont, M.E. & Gorlin, R.J. (1984) Single central incisor in familial holoprosencephaly. *Journal of Pediatrics*, **104**:877–80.

Bodensteiner, J.B. & Shaefer, G.B. (1990) Wide cavum septum pellucidum: a marker of disturbed brain development. *Pediatric Neurology*, 6:391–4.

Chuang, S. & Harwood-Nash, D. (1986) Tumours and cysts. *Neuroradiology*, 28:463–75.

Cubberley, D.A., Jaffe, R.B. & Nixon, G.W. (1982) Sonographic demonstration of Galenic arteriovenous malformation in the neonate. *American Journal of Neuroradiology*, 3:435–9.

Deeg, K.H. & Scharf, J. (1990) Colour Doppler imaging of arteriovenous malformation of the vein of Galen in a newborn. *Neuroradiology*, 32:60–3.

Fakhry, J., Schechter, A., Tenner, M.S. & Reale, M (1985) Cysts of the choroid plexus in neonates: documentation and review of the literature. *Journal of Ultrasound in Medicine*, 4:561–3.

Hernanz-Schulman, M., Dohan, F.C., Jones, T., Cayea, P., Wallman, J. & Teele, R.L. (1985) Sonographic appearance of callosal agenesis. *American Journal of Neuroradiology*, 6:31–368.

Jones, R.W.A., Allan, L.D., Tynan, M.J. & Joseph, M.C. (1982) Ultrasound diagnosis of cerebral arteriovenous malformations in the newborn. *Lancet*, i:102–3.

Joubert, M., Eisenring, J.J. & Robb, J.P. (1969) Familial agenesis of the cerebellar vermis. A syndrome of episodic hyperpnoea, abnormal eye movements, ataxia, and retardation. *Neurology*, 19:813–25.

Keller, M.C., DiPietro, M.A., Teele, R.L., White, S.J., Chawla, H.S., Curtis-Cohen, M. & Blane, C.E. (1987) Periventricular cavitations in the first week of life. *American Journal of Neuroradiology*, 8:291–5.

Lam, A.H. & Villanueva, A.C. (1992) Symptomatic third ventricular choroid plexus cysts. *Pediatric Radiology*, 22:413–16.

Larroche, J.C. (1972) Subependymal pseudocysts in the newborn. *Biology of the Neonate*, 21:170–83.

Leech, R.W. & Shuman, R.M. (1986) Holoprosencephaly and related midline cerebral anomalies. A review. *Journal of Child Neurology*, 1:3–18.

Levene, M.I. (1980) Diagnosis of subependymal pseudocyst with cerebral ultrasound. *Lancet*. ii:210.

Lodeiro, J.G., Feinstein, S.J. & Lodeiro, S.B. (1989) Persisting choroid plexus cysts. *American Journal of Perinatology*, 6:450–2.

Lu, J.H., Emons, D. & Kowalewski, S. (1992) Connatal periventricular pseudocysts in the neonate. *Pediatric Radiology*, 22:55–8.

Lylyk, P., Vinuela, F. & Dion, J.E. (1993) Therapeutic alternatives for vein of Galen vascular malformations. *Journal of Neurosurgery*, 78:438–45.

Pellicer, A., Cabañas, F., Pérez-Higueras, A., Garcia-Alix, A. & Quero, J. (1995) Neural migration disorders studied by cerebral ultrasound and colour Doppler flow imaging. *Archives of Disease in Childhood*, 73: F55–F61.

Pilu, G., Sandri, F., Cerisoli, M., Alvisi, C., Salvioli, G.P. & Bovicelli, L. (1990) Sonographic findings in septo-optic dysplasia in the fetus and newborn infant. *American Journal of Perinatology*, 7:337–9.

Rademaker, K.J., De Vries, L.S. & Barth, P.G. (1993) Subependymal pseudocysts: ultrasound diagnosis and findings at follow up. *Acta Paediatrica Scandinavica*, 82:394–9.

Riebel, T., Nasir, R. & Weber, K. (1992) Choroid plexus cysts: a normal finding on ultrasound. *Pediatric Radiology*, 22:410–12.

Sandri, F., Pilu, G., Cerisoli, M., Bovicelli, L., Alvisi, C. & Salvioli, G.P. (1988) Sonographic diagnosis of agenesis of the corpus callosum in the fetus and newborn infant. *American Journal of Perinatology*. 5:226–31.

Sauerbrei, E.E. & Cooperberg, P.L. (1981) Neonatal brain: sonography of congenital abnormalities. *American Journal of Roentgenology*, **136**:1167–70.

Sauerbrei, E.E. & Cooperberg, P.L. (1983) Cystic tumours of the fetal and neonatal cerebrum: ultrasound and computed tomographic evaluation. *Radiology*, **147**:689–92.

Sheehy-Skeffington, F. (1982) Agenesis of the corpus callosum. *Archives of Disease in Childhood*, **57**:713–14.

Shen, E-Y. & Huang, F.Y. (1985) Subependymal cysts in normal neonates. *Archives of Disease in Childhood*, **60**:1072–4.

Sirry, H.W., Anthony, M.Y. & Whittle, M.J. (1995) Doppler assessment of the fetal and neonatal brain. In *Fetal and Neonatal Neurology and Neurosurgery*, ed. M.I. Levene & R.J. Lilford, pp. 129–44. Edinburgh: Churchill Livingstone.

Sutton, L.N., Bruce, D.A. & Schut, L. (1980) Hydranencephaly versus maximal hydrocephalus: an important clinical distinction. *Neurosurgery*, **6**:35–8.

Teele, R.L., Hernanz-Schulman, M. & Sotrel, A. (1988) Echogenic vasculature in the basal ganglia of neonates: a sonographic sign of vasculopathy. *Radiology*, **169**: 423–7.

Tessler, F.N., Dion, J., Vinuela, F., Perrella, R.R., Duckwiler, G., Hall, T., Boechet, M.I. & Grant, E.G. (1989) Cranial arteriovenous malformations in neonates: color Doppler imaging with angiographic correlation. *American Journal of Radiology*, **153**:1027–30.

Trounce, J.Q., Fagan, D.G, Young, I.D. & Levene, M.I. (1986) Disorders of neuronal migration. *Developmental Medicine and Child Neurology*, **28**:467–1.

Vaksmann, G., Decoulx, E. & Mauran, P. (1989) Evaluation of vein of Galen arteriovenous malformations in newborns by two dimensional ultrasound, pulsed and color Doppler method. *European Journal of Pediatrics*, **148**:510–12.

Volpe, J.J. (1995) Neural tube formation and prosencephalic development. In *Neurology of the Newborn*, ed. J.J. Volpe, pp. 3–52. Philadephia: WB Saunders.

Williams, J., Brodsky, M.C., Griebel, M., Glasier, C.M., Caldwell, D. & Thomas, P. (1993) Septo-optic dysplasia: the clinical insignificance of an absent septum pellucidum. *Developmental Medicine and Child Neurology*, **35**:490–501.

Zorzi, C. & Angonese, I. (1989) Subependymal pseudocysts in the neonate. *European Journal of Pediatrics*, **148**:462–4.

11 *Hypoxic ischaemic encephalopathy*

Introduction

Neonatal encephalopathy presents with fits, change in concious level and altered muscle tone. The most frequent cause is hypoxic ischaemic encephalopathy secondary to birth asphyxia. Other causes of neonatal encephalopathy include inborn metabolic errors, infection and congenital malformations of the brain. Birth depression must be present to support a diagnosis of hypoxic ischaemic encephalopathy, with at least some of the following features:

- Apgar score less than 6 at 5 minutes.
- Delayed spontaneous respiration.
- Cord umbilical arterial blood with a pH less than 7.0.
- Cord umbilical arterial blood with a base deficit of more than −10 mmol/l.
- Fetal distress with a sustained bradycardia (<100 beats per minute).
- Thick meconium staining of the liquor.

Infants with moderately severe hypoxic ischaemic encephalopathy develop refractory convulsions in the first 24–48 hours and have evidence of other organ system damage including renal failure or poor myocardial function. Neuroimaging is required in any neonatal encephalopathic illness, initially to help define the cause and later to identify infants with a poor prognosis. Cranial ultrasound in hypoxic ischaemic encephalopathy can diagnose cerebral oedema and later multicystic encephalomalacia but the changes do not appear early enough to provide a reliable basis for pharmacological intervention. New interventions such as magnesium sulphate or brain cooling (Thordstein *et al.*, 1993; Thoresen *et al.*, 1996) need to be given within a few hours of birth to be effective. Abnormal cerebral blood flow velocity demonstrated with Doppler ultrasound is a good predictor but not until 24 hours after birth (Levene *et al.*, 1989; Eken *et al.*, 1995). Electroencephalography (EEG) is the best early predictor currently available (Hellström-Westas *et al.*, 1995; Eken *et al.*, 1995). A continuous low voltage or flat EEG or burst-supression present on the EEG in the first six hours accurately predicted adverse outcome in 43 of 47 infants (Hellström-Westas *et al.*, 1995).

Cerebral oedema

This is the earliest manifestation of hypoxic ischaemic encephalopathy to appear. Sheehy-Skeffington & Pearse (1983) coined the term 'bright brain' to describe the general increase in echodensity of the cerebral parenchyma seen with an increase in brain water. Similar appearances with loss of normal anatomical landmarks and a snowstorm speckling of the parenchyma were recognised at the same time by Babcock & Ball (1983) and Martin *et al.* (1983). Figure 11.1 shows coronal and parasagittal scans from two cases of hypoxic ischaemic encephalopathy at term. The ventricular cavity is obscured and there is loss of gyral marking throughout both hemispheres. Even the Sylvian fissure, which is usually easily identified, is hard to make out. Whilst this appearance is characteristic of hypoxic ischaemic encephalopathy it is not specific, and a similar ultrasound appearance can be seen in meningitis. The appearances can resolve completely without sequelae so that a diagnosis of cerebral oedema is of no prognostic value.

Thalamic lesions

The thalamus is particularly vulnerable to insult from acute total asphyxia due to high metabolic demand (Myers, 1975; Pasternak, 1991). Shen (1984) read the reports of 'bright brain' in asphyxia and wrote from Taiwan to report a case with a bright thalamus that persisted for at least three months. Later he described finding a bright thalamus in six of 83 cases of birth asphyxia who all developed severe cerebral palsy or died (Shen *et al.*, 1986). Other workers have contributed further cases but the total published experience is still small: Donn *et al.* (1984); Kreusser *et al.* (1984); Voit *et al.* (1987); Hertzberg *et al.* (1987); Cabañas *et al.* (1991); Connolly et al. (1994). An example is given in Fig. 11.2. Recent MRI studies have revealed that thalamic damage may be more common than previously suspected and that a minority of the affected infants develop athetoid cerebral palsy (Rutherford *et al.*, 1992; Martin & Barkovich, 1995). Magnetic resonance proton spectroscopy has confirmed the presence of lactate in the thalamic area which persists for some time (Peden *et al.*, 1993; Groenendaal *et al.*, 1994).

Middle cerebral artery infarction

Other focal lesions such as haemorrhage and particularly middle cerebral artery infarction are well recognised complications of asphyxia (Martin *et al.*, 1983; Levene, 1995). For further discussion see Chapter 6.

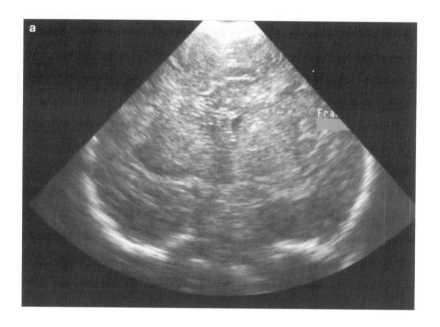

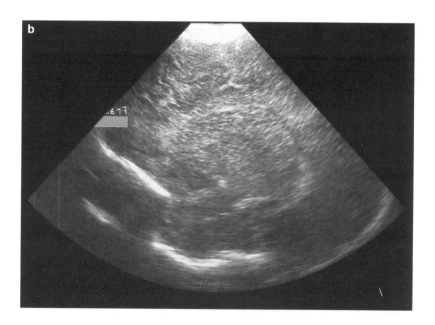

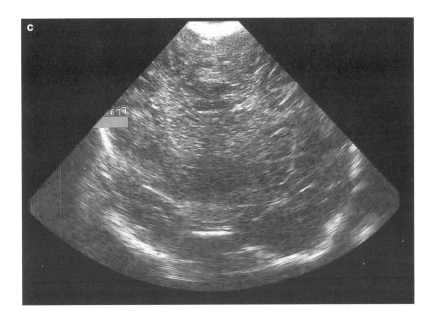

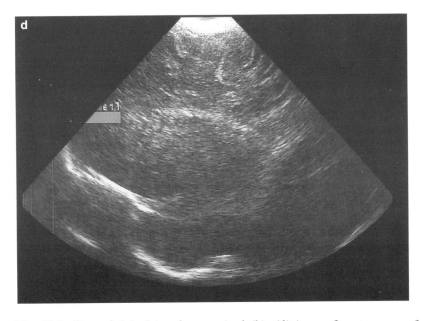

Fig. 11.1. *Coronal (a), (c) and parasagittal (b), (d) images from two cases of hypoxic ischaemic encephalopathy with cerebral oedema.*

199

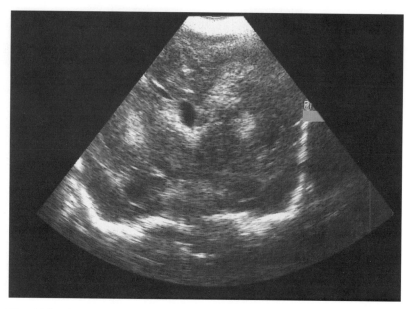

Fig. 11.2. *Coronal image showing echodensity in the region of the thalamus.*

White matter injury and multicystic encephalomalacia

Ultrasound is very useful in the detection of white matter injury due to hypoxia-ischaemia although subtle damage is missed (Hope *et al.*, 1988). The early appearances are more obvious on ultrasound than with CT. Cerebral oedema resolves and may give rise to a generalised patchy, fluffy periventricular echodensity like that seen in Fig. 11.3 or there may be widespread periventricular flares like those illustrated in Fig. 7.12. The areas gradually become cystic over a period of a few weeks. Figure 11.4 shows extensive grade IV periventricular leukomalacia (multicystic encephalomalacia) which developed in a severely asphyxiated term infant whose mother sustained a massive antepartum haemorrhage at home. The early CT scan (Fig. 11.5) confirms the extensive loss of cerebral tissue, which later collapsed to produce external hydrocephalus (Fig. 11.6). A similar case, with extensive multicystic encephalomalacia, is shown in Fig. 11.7. Ultrasound gives a better impression of the extent of the damage than the accompanying CT scan (Fig. 11.8) although MRI confirms the massive loss of cerebral tissue (Fig. 11.9). MRI may prove to be the superior imaging modality for evaluation of hypoxic ischaemic encephalopathy (Volpe, 1995). Preliminary studies suggest that it is more reliable than either ultrasound or CT at detecting basal ganglia damage, focal areas of haemorrhage and infarction and early white matter infarction. However the technique is not widely available and is unsuitable for repeated examinations. Ultrasound evaluation of infants with hypoxic ischaemic encepha-

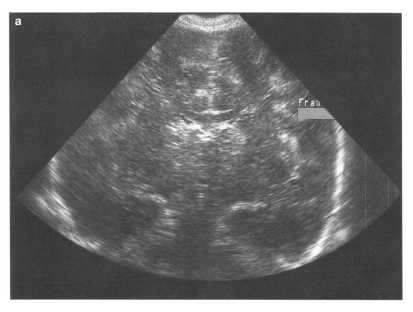

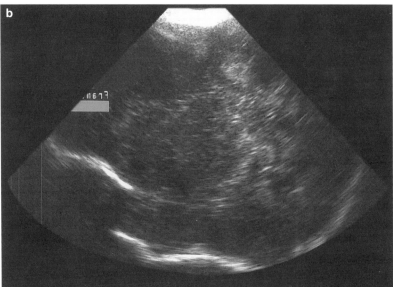

Fig. 11.3. *Coronal (a) and parasagittal (b) images showing fluffy periventricular echodensities in a term infant with birth asphyxia.*

lopathy looks set to continue for the immediate future, and can contribute to our ability to give an accurate prognosis. Infants with encephalopathy should have repeated cranial ultrasound imaging performed in the first week of life, with a CT or MRI scan at about two weeks of age if they survive.

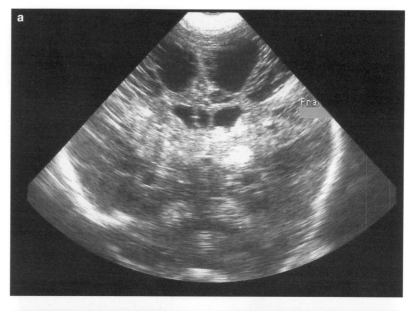

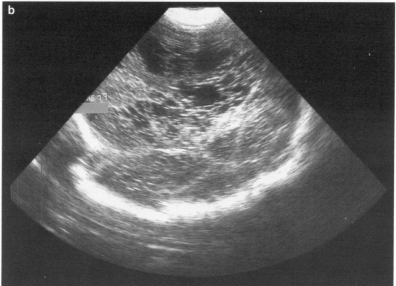

Fig. 11.4. *Extensive multi-cystic encephalomalacia after birth asphyxia at term in coronal (a) and parasagittal (b) images.*

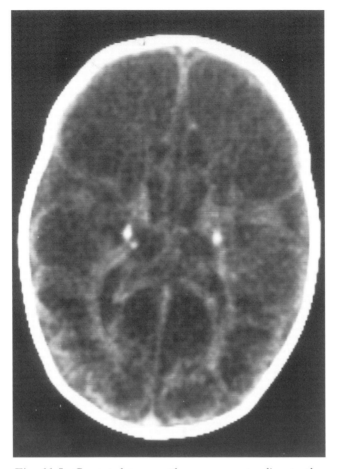

Fig. 11.5. *Computed tomography scan corresponding to the coronal ultrasound image in Fig. 11.4.*

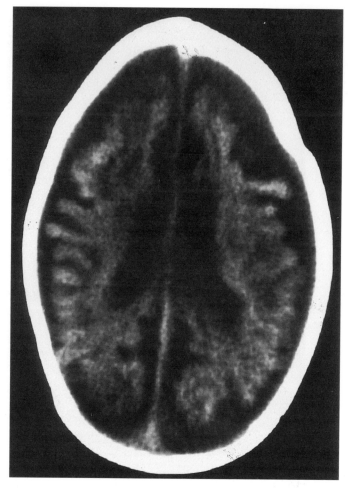

Fig. 11.6. *Late computed tomography scan of the case imagined in Fig. 11.4(a) and Fig. 11.5. The cortex has collapsed to produce external hydrocephalus.*

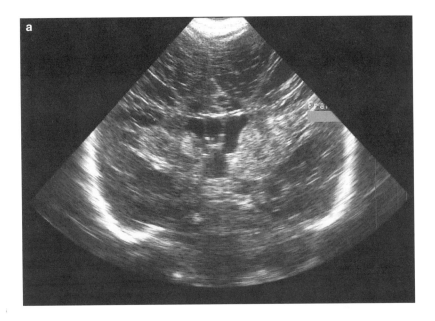

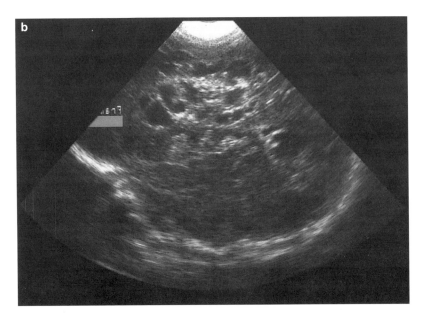

Fig. 11.7. *Coronal (a) and parasagittal (b) ultrasound images showing multi-cystic encephalomalacia.*

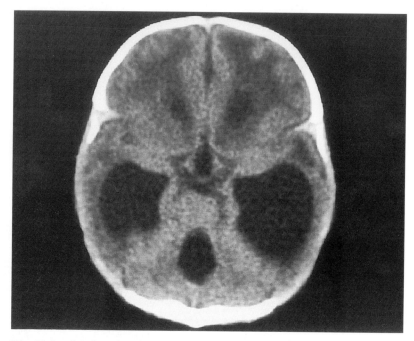

Fig. 11.8. *Axial computed tomography scan of the same case. There is ventriculo-megaly and loss of periventricular white matter.*

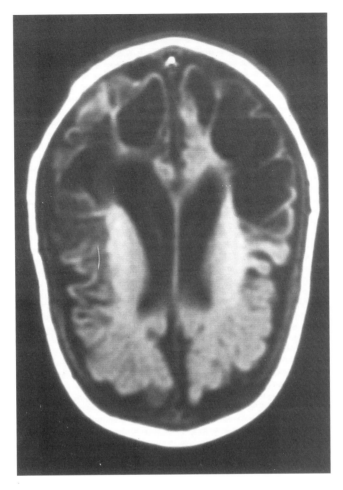

Fig. 11.9. *Magnetic resonance image showing multi-cystic encephalomalacia.*

References

Babcock, D.S. & Ball, W. (1983) Postasphyxial encephalopathy in full term infants: ultrasound diagnosis. *Radiology*, **148**:417–23.

Cabañas, F., Pelicer, A., Pérez-Higueras, A., Garcia-Alix, A., Roche, C. & Quero, J. (1991) Ultrasonographic findings in thalamus and basal ganglia in term asphyxiated infants. *Pediatric Neurology*, **7**:211–15.

Connolly, B., Kelehan, P., O'Brien, N., Gorman, W, Murphy, J.F., King, M. & Donoghue, V. (1994) The echogenic thalamus in hypoxic ischaemic encephalopathy. *Pediatric Radiology*, **24**:268–71.

Donn, S.M., Bowerman, R.A. & DiPietro, M.A. (1984) Sonographic appearance of neonatal thalamic-striatal haemorrhage. *Annals of Neurology*, **16**:361–3.

Eken, P., Toet, MC., Groenendaal, F. & De Vries, L.S. (1995) Predictive value of early neuroimaging, pulsed Doppler and neurophysiology in full term infants with hypoxic-ischaemic encephalopathy. *Archives of Disease in Childhood*, **73**: F75–F80.

Groenendaal, F., Reinier, H.V. & Van Der Grond, J. (1994) Cerebral lactate and N-acetylaspartate/choline ratios in asphyxiated full term neonates demonstrated *in vivo* using magnetic resonance spectroscopy. *Pediatric Research*, **35**:148–51.

Hellström-Westas, L., Rosén, I. & Svenningsen, N.W. (1995) Predictive value of early continuous amplitude integrated EEG recordings on outcome after severe birth asphyxia in full term infants. *Archives of Disease in Childhood*, **72**:F34–F38.

Hertzberg, BS., Pastro, M.E., Needleman, L., Kurtz, A.B. & Rifkin, M.D. (1987) Postasphyxial encephalopathy in term infants. *Journal of Ultrasound in Medicine*, **6**:197–8.

Hope, P.J., Gould, S.J., Howard, S., Hamilton, P.A., Costello, A.M. de L. & Reynolds, E.O.R. (1988) Precision of ultrasound diagnosis of pathologically verified lesions in the brains of very preterm infants. *Developmental Medicine and Child Neurology*, **30**:457–71.

Kreusser, K.L., Schmidt, R.E., Shackleford, G.D. & Volpe, J.J. (1984) Value of ultrasound for identification of acute hemorrhagic necrosis of thalamus and basal ganglia in an asphyxiated term infant. *Annals of Neurology* **16**: 361–3.

Levene, M.I. (1995) The asphyxiated newborn infant. In *Fetal and Neonatal Neurology and Neurosurgery*, ed. M.I. Levene & R.J. Lilford, pp. 405–25. Edinburgh: Churchill Livingstone.

Levene, M.I., Fenton, A.C., Evans, D.H., Archer, L.N.J., Shortland, D.B. & Gibson, N.A. (1989) Severe birth asphyxia and abnormal cerebral blood flow velocity. *Developmental Medicine and Child Neurology*, **31**:427–34.

Martin, D.J., Hill, A., Fitz, C.R., Daneman, A., Havill, D.A. & Becker, L.E. (1983) Hypoxic/ischaemic cerebral injury in the neonatal brain. *Pediatric Radiology*, **13**:307–12.

Martin, E. & Barkovich, A.J. (1995) Magnetic resonance imaging in perinatal asphyxia. *Archives of Disease in Childhood*, **72**:F62–F70.

Myers, R.E. (1975) Four patterns of perinatal brain damage and their conditions of occurrence in primates. *Advances in Neurology*, **10**:223–34.

Pasternak, J.F. (1991) Neonatal asphyxia: vulnerability of the basal ganglia thalamus and brain stem. *Pediatric Neurology*, **7**:147–9.

Peden, C.J., Rutherford, M.A., Sargentoni, J. Cox, I.J., Bryant, D.J. & Dubowitz, L.M.S. (1993) Proton spectroscopy of the neonatal brain following hypoxic-ischaemic injury. *Developmental Medicine and Child Neurology*, **35**:502–10.

Rutherford, M.A., Pennock, J.M., Murdoch-Eaton, D.M., Cowan, F. & Dubowitz, L.M.S. (1992) Athetoid cerebral palsy with cysts in the putamen after hypoxic-ischaemic encephalopathy. *Archives of Disease in Childhood*, **67**:846–50.

Sheehy-Skeffington, F. & Pearse, R.G. (1983) The 'bright brain'. *Archives of Disease in Childhood*, **58**:509–11.

Shen, E.-Y. (1984) The bright thalamus. *Archives of Disease in Childhood*, **59**:695.

Shen, E.-Y., Huang, C.C., Chyou, S.C., Hung, H.Y., Hsu, C.H. & Huang, F.Y. (1986) Sonographic finding of the bright thalamus. *Archives of Disease in Childhood*, **61**:1096–9.

Thordstein, M., Bågenholm, R., Thiringer, K. & Kjellmer, I. (1993) Scavengers of free radicals in combination with magnesium ameliorate perinatal hypoxic-ischaemic brain damage in the rat. *Pediatric Research*, **34**:23–6.

Thoresen, M., Bågenholm, R., Løberg, E. M., Apricena, F. & Kjellmer, I. (1996) Posthypoxic cooling of neonatal rats provides protection against brain injury. *Archives of Disease in Childhood*, **74**:F3–F9.

Voit, T., Lemburg, P., Neven, E., Lumenta, C. & Stork, W. (1987) Damage of thalamus and basal ganglia in asphyxiated full term neonates. *Neuropaediatrics*, **18**:176–81.

Volpe, J.J. (1995) Hypoxic-ischaemic encephalopathy. In *Neurology of the Newborn*, ed J.J. Volpe, pp. 314–69. Philadephia: W.B. Saunders.

12 *Cranial ultrasound imaging and prognosis*

Introduction

'Our ability to assess and report the outcome of surviving very low birthweight infants has lagged behind our willingness to resuscitate them' (Escobar *et al.*, 1991).

This remains true, although considerable research endeavour has been directed at the evaluation of neonatal cranial ultrasound as a proxy for neurodevelopmental outcome. The following factors have helped to drive these efforts:

- Cost and difficulty of mounting large follow-up studies.
- Length of time taken to obtain a result from follow-up studies.
- Parental requests for early prediction of outcome.
- Curiosity about the epidemiology and natural history of intracranial lesions.
- Pressure for quality control and audit.
- Hope of defining a high risk group who may benefit from early intervention.

These ambitious demands would be difficult for any technique to meet. I hope to give enough information to enable the reader to judge how well cranial ultrasound can achieve these aims.

Background

Epidemiology of handicap in preterm survivors

The high prevalence of neurological impairment in survivors of preterm birth remains a cause for concern. Disabilities which are more common include spastic diplegia, hemplegia and quadriplegia with and without neurodevelopmental delay or poor vision. The prevalence of cerebral palsy amongst babies born in the Mersey region between 1966 and 1977 was 1.5 per 1000 livebirths overall, but 15 per 1000 for those with birthweight <1500 g (Pharoh *et al.*, 1987). The incidence in the latter group reached a peak of 60 per 1000 in 1984 (Fig. 12.1a; Pharoh *et al.*, 1990). Equally high rates have been reported from other population-based registries in Western Australia (Fig. 12.1b), Sweden and California (Hagberg *et al.*, 1989; Grether *et al.*, 1992; Stanley & Watson, 1992; Hagberg *et al.*, 1993).

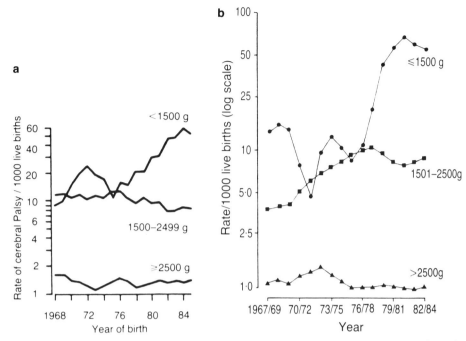

Fig. 12.1. *Incidence of cerebral palsy by birthweight group in Western Australia (a) and in the Mersey region of the UK (b). (Reproduced with permission from (a): Stanley & Watson, 1992; (b): Pharoh et al., 1990.)*

Impairment of vision or hearing can also result in significant handicap for a child. Poor school performance due to clumsiness, epilepsy, language disorder, behavioural problems or short attention span affects 20–40% of surviving very low birthweight (VLBW) children without major handicap (Calame *et al.*, 1986; Levene *et al.*, 1992; Scottish Low Birthweight Study Group, 1992a; Pharoh *et al.*, 1994). Attempts to summarise the vast follow-up literature in order to draw unified conclusions are hampered by many inconsistencies (Mutch *et al.*, 1989; Chalmers & Altman, 1995). Differences between studies include:

- Lack of agreed criteria for diagnosis of cerebral palsy or developmental delay.
- Differences in the definition of major and minor handicap.
- Wide range of age at acertainment.
- Lack of blinding.
- Variable and often large numbers of lost children.
- Hospital-based rather than geographical cohorts.
- Gestational age or birthweight cut-offs to define cohorts.

Differences in definition and age at acertainment accounted for much of the variation in the incidence of cerebral palsy seen in the 85 studies subjected to a meta-analysis by Escobar *et al.* (1991). The mean rate was 7.7% with 95% confidence intervals from 5.3 to 9.0 and a range from

211

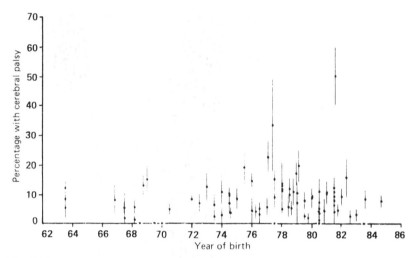

Fig. 12.2. *Meta-analysis of studies reporting cerebral palsy by year of birth cohort. The vertical axis represents the reported incidence for each of 85 eligible cohorts. The horizontal axis indicates the midpoint of the period of enrolment. Each bar represents the mean (SD) rate of a single cohort of subjects. (Reproduced with permission from Escobar et al., 1991.)*

0 to 50 (Fig. 12.2). Cerebral palsy was diagnosed at the age of two years in 7.9% of a geographical cohort of over a thousand children whose birthweight was <2 kg (Pinto-Martin *et al.*, 1995). A further 6.7% had non-disabling mild spastic diplegia. Similar figures of 7.6% disabled and 5.7% with neurological signs were reported from a geographical population of 908 babies <1750 g (Scottish Low Birthweight Study Group 1992b). In 1980 the World Health Organisation tried to reduce confusion by defining impairment, disability and handicap (Table 12.1). Stewart (1992) has suggested useful guidelines for future outcome studies which should reach a minimum standard to be acceptable for publication. She has also devised a structured method for recording the results of neurological examination (Amiel-Tison & Stewart, 1989).

Lesions which predict disability

Cohort screening of asymptomatic VLBW infants with cranial ultrasound has uncovered a high incidence of lesions involving the periventricular zone. Although damage to pre-myelin cells abundant in this region provides a convenient explanation for the high prevalence of cerebral palsy, a causal relationship remains to be proven. Cysts in the parenchyma and cerebral atrophy indicate loss of white matter and are the strongest predictors yet found for cerebral palsy (Paneth *et al.*, 1994; Pinto-Martin *et al.*, 1995). Delayed myelination has been confirmed with later MRI studies, suggesting that the cysts are markers of even more diffuse injury to oligodendroglia (van de Bor *et al.*, 1989a, 1992; Guit *et al.*, 1990; De Vries *et*

Table 12.1. *World Health Organisation definitions of impairment, disability and handicap*

Impairment
　Any loss or abnormality of psychological or anatomical structure or function: in principle, impairments represent disturbances at organ level.

Disability
　Any restriction or lack (resulting from an impairment) of ability to perform an activity in the manner or within the range considered normal for a human being. A disability thus reflects the consequence of an impairment in terms of functional performance and activity by an individual.

Handicap
　A disadvantage for a given individual resulting from an impairment or disability that limits or prevents the fulfilment of a role that is normal (depending on age, sex and social and cultural factors). Handicap thus reflects interaction with the surroundings and is a difficult outcome to use for comparison as it depends on attitudes within the family and society to disability.

al., 1993). Most studies are in remarkable agreement, showing a fivefold increase in the risk of cerebral palsy following ultrasound diagnosis of any parenchymal lesion, and a fifteen-fold increase in the presence of bilateral occipital periventricular leukomalacia. Accumulated experience is still relatively meagre, however, and the predictions have wide confidence intervals due to the small numbers of cases. Clinicians and parents vary in the degree of certainty which they require in order to base a decision on any test result. Cranial ultrasound cannot yet satisfy all these different and exacting requirements. Prediction of learning difficulties, which in some cases may be due to lesser degrees of white matter damage, is still imprecise (Levene *et al.*, 1992). Visual handicap can be accurately predicted from ultrasound abnormalities (Hungerford *et al.*, 1986; Scher *et al.*, 1989; Weisglas-Kuperus *et al.*, 1993; Eken *et al.*, 1994; Pike *et al.*, 1994).

White matter damage carries a high probability of cerebral palsy but by no means all cases in VLBW survivors have early ultrasound abnormalities. All but 7 of 45 children so afflicted had periventricular cysts or echodensity (Graziani *et al.*, 1992). In contrast, of 91 children with a major handicap at 18 months, 41 had normal ultrasound findings in the neonatal period (Rennie unpub. data). Prolonged artificial ventilation for bronchopulmonary dysplasia may be a factor in those without obvious intracranial pathology (Wheater & Rennie, 1994; Pinto-Martin *et al.*, 1995). Inadequate or incorrect nutrition at a critical period may be another (Lucas *et al.*, 1990). Preterm male infants have double the risk of cerebral palsy than female preterm infants (Brothwood *et al.*, 1986; Rennie *et al.*, 1996). A normal scan is not therefore a guarantee of a normal outcome, although the chances are about 90% (Ng & Dear, 1990).

213

Use of predictive ability in passive euthanasia

In rare cases the intracranial abnormality is so severe that, in the light of current knowledge, major handicap seems certain. In the unusual circumstance that this information is available at a time when the infant is critically ill and is ventilator dependent there may be grounds for discussing withdrawal of life support with the parents. One example would be extensive bilateral parenchymal echodensities, although very few preterm infants survive an intracranial insult of this magnitude however aggressive the management. The mortality rate of infants with large unilateral parenchymal lesions was 80% (Guzzetta *et al.*, 1986). Bilateral occipital cystic periventricular leukomalacia, currently the most certain harbinger of a poor neurological prognosis, cannot be diagnosed until several weeks of age unless of prenatal origin. In my view, cranial ultrasound alone cannot be used to justify euthanasia in an otherwise stable infant; the predictions are not certain enough and the natural history has not yet reached a 'steady state'. Often, however, a significant cerebral lesion co-exists with severe respiratory failure, prolonged hypotension, renal failure and circulatory shock. In this situation the ultrasound findings combine with the poor prognosis of acidosis and hypoxia to make the withdrawal of intensive care justified. In most such cases death is inevitable and withdrawal of care merely gives the parents and doctors some control over the timing of the event in order to allow privacy and dignity. That cranial ultrasound is used more liberally in this way in the Netherlands has been discussed (Hellema 1992), and is suggested by the high mortality (27%) and low incidence of major handicap (5%) in Dutch VLBW infant survivors (Van de Bor *et al.*, 1989b). Stephenson & Barbor (1995) provide an excellent entry into the debate on the ethics, landmark medico-legal rulings and quality of life arguments which surround infant euthanasia.

The future

The intense interest in 'telling the future' (Levene 1990) with cranial ultrasound lies in the desire to identify those children who are destined to be handicapped at a time when the brain has unique plasticity (Wigglesworth, 1989; Farmer & Harrison, 1991). In future it may be possible to influence the inevitable, programmed cell death which is part of normal brain development (Janowsky, 1986; Gluckman, 1992). Glutamate released from dying neurones is toxic to differentiating neuroglia and this can be prevented *in vitro* with free radical scavengers (Oka *et al.*, 1993). New synapses are formed during the neonatal period and can be redirected using cytokines and growth factors (Patterson *et al.*, 1993). Until the hopes of reproducing these results *in vivo* are realised, prediction of handicap can merely deflate parental optimism and needs sensitive handling. Some parents appreciate the early warning; others do not. There is scant evidence that early intervention with physiotherapy or sensory stimulation is ben-

214

eficial (Achenbach *et al.*, 1993), so that it is difficult to justify cohort scanning of VLBW infants on the basis that the prognosis will be changed for the worse in 10%. Trends are useful for audit and monitoring the effect of changes in practice – a reduction in GMH-IVH due to antenatal steroids in this way has been detected (Maher *et al.*, 1994; Rennie *et al.*, 1996). In future it may be possible to compare performance with units with a similar case-mix via a suitable clinical risk score (International Neonatal Network, 1993).

Prognosis after specific cranial ultrasound diagnosis

Normal cranial ultrasound image

A meta-analysis of the results of follow-up of 992 preterm babies with normal cranial ultrasound scans revealed that 875 (88%) had a normal outcome (Ng & Dear, 1990). The babies were studied in 10 centres throughout Europe, North America and Australia. Table 12.2 shows the numbers of infants and type of follow-up carried out and extends the observations with data from subsequent studies. The outcome of over 3500 preterm infants enrolled in 18 studies has now been reported: over 2000 of these infants had a normal scan and of these 89% were normal at follow-up. Not all the early researchers followed up an entire cohort (Palmer *et al.*, 1982; Graziani *et al.*, 1985). In the research published since 1986 complete cohort studies have been usual. Studies such as those of Williams *et al.* (1987); Beverley *et al.* (1990) and Bozynski *et al.* (1990), which followed up less than 66% of the original cohort or examined the infants at less than one year of age, have not been included in Table 12.2, nor have later non-cohort studies (Goldstein *et al.*, 1989). Some groups have slightly enlarged and extended the duration of follow-up for the original cohort (Van de Bor *et al.*, 1988, 1993; Kitchen *et al.*, 1985, 1990; Fawer & Calame, 1987, 1991) without changing the message, and others enlarged the cohort but stopped following up infants with normal ultrasound scans (Graziani *et al.*, 1986).

The risk of a significant disability, which is often a major handicap, is very small for a preterm infant who has a normal cranial ultrasound scan in the neonatal period, particularly if this is repeated before discharge. From Table 12.2 it can be seen that only 128 children with a normal scan had a major handicap (6%: 95% confidence intervals from 5 to 7). The results of this 'meta-analysis' should be treated with caution, however, as the original cohorts were not strictly comparable. In some of these cases the diagnosis was not cerebral palsy, but visual handicap or developmental delay. The numbers of infants in Table 12.2 do not add up because some died and some had minor handicaps which were not always reported. Figure 12.3 shows the percentage of major handicaps wih 95% confidence intervals for each study arranged by year of cohort entry. The relatively high risk in the Cambridge, UK cohort (Rennie, unpub. data) probably

215

Table 12.2. *Summary of reports containing information on outcome of preterm infants with normal cranial ultrasound scan*

First author / total cohort size	Year of cohort	No. with normal scan/no. seen	Gestation (wks)	Birthweight (g)	Follow-up details	Normal scan only			
						normal outcome (n)	normal outcome (%) and (95% CI)	major handicap (n)	major handicap (%) and (95% CI)
Palmer (1982) not cohort study	1979–80	14/39	27–34	790–2500	12 mo, Griffiths 96% traced	14	93% (66–100)	0	0% (0–23)
Graziani (1985) not cohort study	?	21/53	<33	<1501	20–30 mo, Bayley 100% traced	15	71% (48–89)	2	9% (1–30)
Catto-Smith (1985) n=56	1981	11/31	23–28	567–1378	24 mo, Bayley 95% traced	10	91% (59–100)	1	1% (0–41)
Kitchen (1985) n=227	1980–81	105/148	>23	<1500	24 mo, Bayley 95% traced	93	89% (82–95)	12	11% (5–17)
TeKolste (1985) not cohort study	1980–81	43/72	<32	<1500	22 mo, Bayley 73% traced	29	67% (51–81)	5	12% (4–25)
Szymonowicz (1986) n=50	1982	16/32	24–32	430–1250	24 mo, Bayley 100% traced	16	100% (79–100)	0	0% (0–21)
Greisen (1986) n=121	?	57/114	30±1.6 (SD)	<1500	24 mo, Denver clin. exam. 100%	51	90% (78–96)	5	9% (3–19)
Cooke (1987a) n=798	1980–84	333/524		<1501	24–60 mo, clin. exam. 100%	314	94% (91–96)	19	6% (3–9)
Fawer (1987, 1991) n=112	?	61/93	<34	1554±384	18 mo, Griffiths 5y neurol. exam. 82%	61	100% (94–100)	0	0% (0–6)
Graham (1987) n=200	?	64/156		<1501	18 mo, Griffiths 99% traced	61	95% (87–99)	3	5% (1–13)
Stewart (1987) n=485	1979–81	184/342	24–32	535–2500	12 mo, Griffiths 96% traced	166	90% (85–94)	8	4% (2–8)
Bozynski (1988) n=152	?	67/116	28.7	<1201	12–18 mo, Milani 66% traced	42	63% (50–74)	3	4% (1–12)
Tudehope (1989) n=218	1983–85	96/147	28	<1500	24 mo, Griffiths 99% traced	86	90% (82–95)	10	10% (5–18)

Study								
Fazzi (1992) n=203	?	53/148	24–36	<1501	1–3 yr clin. exam. Bayley 83% seen	49	92% (82–98)	4	7% (2–18)
Weisglas–Kuperus (1992) n=114	1985–86	22/79	<36	<1500	90% seen at 3.5y neurological exam. of Touwen	20	91% (71–99)	2	9% (1–29)
Van de Bor (1993) n=484	1983	234/304	<32	<1500	Questionnaire+exam 100% follow-up	177	76% (70–81)	13	5% (3–9)
Pinto-Martin (1995) n=1105	?	565/727		<2000	2 y clin. exam. 86% traced	531	94% (92–96)	0	0% (0–1)
Rennie (unpub. data) n=658	1985–92	344/470	23–38	<1501	18 mo, Bayley 86% traced	303	88% (85–92)	41	12% (8–15)
Totals*		2290 with normal scan				2037	89% (88–90)	128	6% (5–7)

*NB The totals from the outcome columns and the total number of infants with the ultrasound appearance in column 2 do not add up in this or subsequent tables in this chapter. This is due to late deaths, and varying numbers of infants with minor handicaps who have not been included.

CI: confidence intervals.

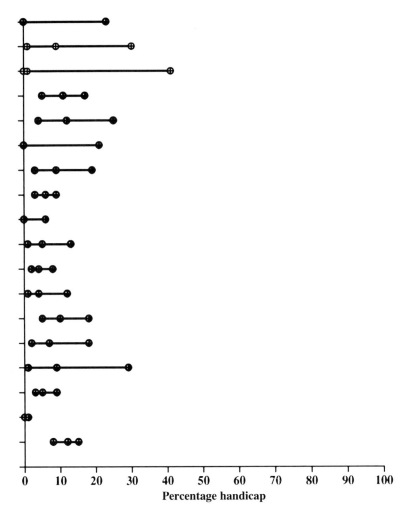

Fig. 12.3. *Risk of major handicap in very low birthweight infants with a normal cranial ultrasound scan shown as a percentage, with bars representing 95% confidence intervals from Table 12.2, arranged in the same order (first at the top).*

reflects the increasingly low gestational age of current survivors. If this trend is confirmed it may mean that cranial ultrasound will become less useful as a predictor of outcome in future.

Germinal matrix haemorrhage (GMH)

There is consistent agreement that isolated germinal matrix haemorrhage is not associated with an increased risk of handicap (Table 12.3). Several studies report outcome of 'uncomplicated periventricular haemorrhage' where this is defined as increased echodensity within the lateral ventricle but without parenchymal echodensity or ventriculomegaly. This early

Table 12.3. *Summary of reports containing information on outcome of preterm infants with subependymal haemorrhage (SEH) alone*

First author, total cohort size	No. with SEH/ No. seen	Gestation (wks)	Birthweight (g)	Follow-up details	SEH alone diagnosed with ultrasound	
					normal outcome (n)	major handicap (n)
Palmer (1982) not cohort study	12/39	27–34	790–2500	12 mo, Griffiths 96% traced	12	0
Catto-Smith (1985) n=56	14/31	23–28	567–1378	24 mo, Bayley 95% traced	12	2
Kitchen (1985) n=227	20/148	>23	500–1500	24 mo, Bayley 95% traced	17	3
TeKolste (1985) not cohort study	14/72	<32	<1500	22 mo, Bayley 73% traced	12	6
Szymonowicz (1986) n=50	4/32	24–32	430–1250	24 mo, Bayley 100% traced	4	0
Cooke (1987a) n=798	73/524		<1501	24–60 mo, clin. exam. 100%	59	1
Tudehope (1989) n=218	31/162	28	<1500	24 mo, Griffiths 99% traced	31	0
Totals	168 with SEH				147 (88%) (95% CI 82–92)	12 (7%) (95% CI 4–12)

CI: confidence intervals

ultrasound finding is also associated with a good chance of normal outcome (Table 12.4). Subependymal pseudocysts appear like strings of beads which lie along the floor of the lateral ventricle. They are a congenital lesion that can be associated with other congenital abnormalities but which have a good prognosis (Rademaker *et al.*, 1993).

Enlarged cerebral ventricles

Enlargement of the lateral ventricles, often defined as more than 4 mm above the 97th centile of Levene (1981), is a frequent finding in preterm neonates who have sustained GMH-IVH. It is important to distinguish ventricular dilatation due to cerebral atrophy from progressive hydrocephalus as a consequence of raised cerebrospinal fluid pressure. Cerebral atrophy is associated with an irregularly shaped ventricle and there may be evidence of loss of white matter in the parenchyma. Head growth is normal or reduced, the fontanelle tension is lax and there are no symptoms of raised intracranial pressure. Progressive hydrocephalus tends to begin with trigonal enlargement and is associated with increased occipitofrontal circumference and suture divarification. The cerebrospinal fluid pressure is raised, usually above 10 cm, and there may be symptoms such as apnoea or vomiting. Pressure alone cannot be used to predict progression as some cases who eventually require surgical drainage have low pressure (Kaiser & Whitelaw, 1985), but there is a tendency for progressive disease to be associated with a cerebrospinal fluid pressure above the upper limit of normal – about 7.8 cm cerebrospinal fluid (6 mmHg or 0.8 kPa).

The natural history of ventriculomegaly is that about 50–60% will have progressive hydrocephalus and require surgical intervention, usually the insertion of a ventriculo-peritoneal shunt (Allan *et al.*, 1982; Dykes *et al.*, 1989; Ventriculomegaly Trial Group, 1990). This is usually a slow progression over several weeks although a few unfortunate infants develop rapidly progressive hydrocephalus. Intervention is indicated for rapidly increasing head circumference of more than 2 cm per week, symptoms or an intracranial pressure above 15 cm cerebrospinal fluid. Repeated aspiration of cerebrospinal fluid in the early period after diagnosis cannot prevent the need for surgical drainage or the subsequent neurological deficit (Ventriculomegaly Trial Group, 1990, 1994). The collaborative ventriculomegaly trial enrolled 157 infants from 15 centres who were followed to 30 months by a single observer. Infants were randomly allocated to groups receiving either repeated early drainage or conservative management; there was no difference in outcome at one year or 30 months; only 11 of 112 were normal, underlining the poor prognosis for this group. In Table 12.5, I have summarised the outcome for infants with ventriculomegaly who do not have associated parenchymal lesions, and in Table 12.6 for those with shunted hydrocephalus due to lack of detail in the studies published to date. Cooke (1987b), and the Ventriculomegaly Trial Group (1990,1994) found that the outcome was worse for infants with fits or parenchymal

Table 12.4. *Summary of reports containing information on outcome of preterm infants with uncomplicated GMH–IVH*

First author, total cohort size	No. with finding/No. seen	Gestation (wks)	Birthweight (g)	Follow-up details	Uncomplicated *GMH–IVH*			
					normal outcome (n)	normal outcome (%) and (95% CI)	major handicap (n)	major handicap (%) and (95% CI)
Palmer (1982) not cohort study	14/39	27–34	790–2500	12 mo, Griffiths 96% traced	14	100% (77–100)	0	0% (0–23)
Catto-Smith (1985) n=56	17/31	<28	567–1378	24 mo, Bayley 95% traced	9	53% (28–77)	8	47% (23–72)
TeKolste (1985) not cohort study	27/72	<32	<1500	22 mo, Bayley 73% traced	16	59%(39–78)	8	30% (14–50)
Graziani (1985) not cohort study	22/53	<33	<1501	20–30 mo, Bayley 100% traced	16	73% (50–89)	3	14% (3–35)
Greisen (1986) n=121	26/114	30±1.6 (SD)	<1500	24 mo Denver, clin. exam. 100%	25	96% (80–100)	1	4% (0–20)
Stewart (1987) n=485	101/342	24–32	535–2500	12 mo Griffiths 96% traced	97	96% (90–99)	4	4% (1–10)
Graham 1987 n=200	74/156		<1501	18 mo, Griffiths 99% traced	74	100% (95–100)	0	0% (0–5)
Tudehope (1989) n=218	38/162	28	<1500	24 mo, Griffiths 99% traced	26	68% (51–82)	2	5% (1–18)
Kitchen (1990) n=227	33/139	>23	500–1500	24 mo, Bayley 95% traced	31	94% (80–99)	2	6% (1–20)
Bozynski (1990) n=155	12/51	AGA	<1251	50% seen Dubowitz neurological exam	5	42% (15–72)	6	50% (21–79)
Fawer (1991) n=112	17/93	<34	1554±384	5yrs Touwen neurological exam 82% traced	17	100% (80–100)	0	0% (0–20)
Weisglas-Kuperus (1992) n=114	20/79	<36	<1500	90% seen 3.5y neurological exam of Touwen	19	95% (75–100)	1	5% (0–25)
Fazzi (1992) n=203	26/148	24–36	<1501	1–3 y clin exam. Bayley 83% seen	23	88% (70–98)	3	11% (2–30)
Van de Bor 1993 n=484	50/304	<32	<1500	Questionnaire + exam 100% follow up	45	90% (78–97)	5	10% (3–22)
Pinto-Martin (1995) n=1105	149/727		<2000	2y clinical exam 86% traced	102	69% (61–76)	37	25% (18–32)
Totals	626 cases				519	83% (80–86)	80	13% (10–15)

CI: confidence intervals; SD: standard deviation; AGA: apppropriate gestational age; GMH-IVH: germinal matrix haemorrhage–intraventricular haemorrhage.

Table 12.5. *Summary of reports containing information on outcome of infants with isolated, non-progressive ventriculomegaly alone*

First author, total cohort size	No. with finding/ No. seen	Gestation (wks)	Birthweight (g)	Follow-up details	Isolated ventriculomegaly	
					normal outcome	major handicap
Palmer (1982) not cohort study	9/39	27–34	790–2500	12 mo, Griffiths 96% traced	1	5
Allan (1984) n=268	14/268	<35		all traced, Denver	12	2
Graziani (1985) no. not given	6/53	<33	<1501	20–30 mo, Bayley 100% traced	6	0
Greisen (1986) n=121	21/114	30±1.6 (SD)	<1500	24 mo Denver, clin exam 100%	15	6
Stewart (1987) n=485	41/342	24–32	535–2500	12 mo Griffiths 96% traced	30	11
Cooke (1987a) n=798	40/524		<1501	24–60 mo, clin exam, 100%	32	8
Shankaran (1989) n=111	10/111	<35	<1500	12–30 mo Bayley all seen	7	3
Kitchen (1990) n=227	2/148	>23	500–1500	24 mo, Bayley 95% traced	1	1
Weisglas-Kuperus (1992) n=114	30/79	<36	<1500	90% seen at 3.5y Touwen exam.	16	14
Ventriculomegaly Trial Group (1994)	53	28±3	<1500	only 4 cases lost 30 mo Griffiths	6	26
Totals	226 cases				126 (56%) (95% CI 50–63)	76 (34%) (95% CI 28–40)

CI: confidence intervals; SD: standard deviation.

Table 12.6. Summary of reports containing information on outcome of infants with shunted hydrocephalus

First author	No. of cases	Gestation (wks)	Birthweight (g)	Follow-up details	Shunted hydrocephalus	
					normal outcome (n)	major handicap (n)
Palmer (1982)	1	27–34	790–2500	12 mo, Griffiths	1	0
Leichty (1983)	13	34±4.1	2100±1090	12 mo, Bayley	8	5
Allan (1984)	3	<35		Denver	0	3
Boynton (1986)	50	30±2	1266±303	Bayley	7	26
Cooke (1987b)	54		<2500	24–60 mo, clin. exam.	13	37
Etches (1987)	29	25–37	<2000	18 mo, Bayley	5	11
Hislop (1988)	19	25–39	<2740	variable	4	12
Shankaran (1989)	23	<35	<1500	12–30 mo, Bayley	8	11
Fazzi (1992)	6	24–36	<1501	1–3 y clin. exam.	3	3
Fernell (1993)	42	<34	<2500	variable	7	32
Totals	240				56 (24% CI 18–30)	140 (59% CI 53–65)

CI: confidence intervals

echodensities. Shankaran *et al.* (1989) have pointed out the high revision rate required by preterm infants – in this series, 18 children had 82 revisions between them and this worsened the prognosis.

Periventricular leukomalacia

There is no doubt that cystic periventricular leukomalacia is the most powerful predictor of cerebral palsy amongst the neonatal cranial ultrasound lesions so far described. In many cohort follow-up studies almost all the cases of cerebral palsy had bilateral occipital leukomalacia in the neonatal period (Graham *et al.*, 1987; Pidcock *et al.*, 1990). Cysts involving more than one zone also have a poor prognosis (Shortland *et al.*, 1988). Earlier studies, reporting an association between ventricular dilatation and adverse outcome (Table 12.6) probably included some undiagnosed cases of periventricular leukomalacia due to poor resolution of the older, 5 Mhz scanheads. Single cysts and cysts confined to the frontal region appear to have a better outcome than multiple bilateral occipital cysts, where the outlook is universally dismal. Too few studies have reported the outcome of anterior or central cysts to make it possible to give a confident prediction of a good outcome, although most of the reported survivors with single unilateral cysts or cysts confined to the frontal zone are normal at follow-up (Graham *et al.*, 1987; Shortland *et al.*, 1988; Fawer & Calame, 1991; Fazzi *et al.*, 1992). There is even less information about the ultrasound appearance of transient echodensity in the periventricular zone which does not progress to cystic change. Several groups have suggested that this appearance might indicate a minor degree of damage to the pre-myelin cells and have shown an increased incidence of neurological signs and/or clumsiness in later childhood (De Vries *et al.*, 1988, 1993; Appleton *et al.*, 1990; Levene *et al.*, 1992; Jongmans *et al.*, 1993). Table 12.7 summarises the outcome for 124 cases of bilateral occipital periventricular leukomalacia – 93% of the survivors are seriously handicapped. The predominant diagnosis at follow-up was cerebral palsy, either spastic quadriplegia or diplegia. Developmental delay was less often observed. Some large studies have been excluded because it was not possible to distinguish the outcome for different types of periventricular leukomalacia (Sinha *et al.*, 1990), or no late scan appearances were included (Whitaker *et al.*, 1990) or because several conditions were 'lumped' together (Greisen *et al.*, 1986; Bozynski *et al.*, 1990; Pinto-Martin *et al.*, 1995). Thirty-one of 45 cases from a cohort of 497 with cystic periventricular leukomalacia, where the cysts were greater than 3mm in size, developed cerebral palsy but the location of the cysts was not further defined (Graziani *et al.*, 1992). There is duplication of cases in some series and where this occurs only the latest report is included in Table 12.7 (De Vries *et al.*, 1985, 1987; Graham *et al.*, 1987). Fortunately periventricular leukomalacia of this severity is rare, occurring in only 2% of VLBW infants. The challenge for the next decade is to understand the factors which render infants vulnerable to damage to the

Table 12.7. *Cases of bilateral occipital periventricular leukomalacia and their outcome*

Author	Cohort size, details	No. cases	No. with CP
Weindling (1985)	124 <1500 or <34w	8	8
De Vries (1987)	676 <34 weeks	12	4 died; 6 CP; 2 <9mo
Graham (1987)	n=200 <1500g	8	8
Fawer (1987)	n=112 <1500g	5	5
Cooke (1987a)	n=798 <1500g	24	21
Monset-Couchard (1988)	n=471 <1500g	6	6
Hansen (1989)	n≃1600 mostly <1500g	16	16
Pidcock (1990)	n=288	20	18
Weisglas-Kuperus (1992)	n=79 <1500g	2	1
Pierrat (1993)	not given; 33 cases in 2y	9	1 died; 8 CP
Fazzi (1994)	n=299 <32 weeks	14	14
Total	>4373	124	111

CP: cerebral palsy

developing oligodendroglia, in order to reduce this devastating complication of prematurity. Antenatal white matter damage is perhaps more common than we suspect and was demonstrated with careful neuropathological examination in 20% of a series of perinatal autopsies (Gaffney *et al.*, 1994). There is an association with intrauterine growth retardation and chorioamnionitis (Sinha *et al.*, 1990; Gaffney *et al.*, 1994).

Porencephalic cyst secondary to parenchymal haemorrhage

The earlier literature reporting outcome of 'grade IV periventricular haemorrhage' must now be reinterpreted in the light of knowledge about the importance of distinguishing cases of periventricular leukomalacia involving extensive loss of myelin from single porencephalic cysts. Rereading the studies in the light of current thinking serves only to highlight the fact that many of the infants had multiple cystic lesions. I have therefore not attempted to form a table. Volpe's group were amongst the first to realise that all parenchymal lesions were not the same, although their classification did not illuminate the problem at the time (Guzetta *et al.*, 1986). Cooke (1987a) claimed that a porencephalic cyst was a better predictor of cerebral palsy than periventricular leukomalacia but he made a retrospective reclassification of scans originally made in the early 1980s by those who were not aware of leukomalacia at the outset. There is no doubt that

unilateral parenchymal echodensities which evolve into isolated single porencephalic cysts can give rise to no neurological signs at all (De Vries *et
al.*, 1985; Kitchen *et al.*, 1990; Blackman *et al.*, 1991). These children are
rare, but sufficiently frequently reported to make the outcome of porence-
phaly much less certain than that of periventricular leukomalacia. Complex
pathology is a further confounder – there were only three survivors with
porencephalic cysts from a cohort of 200 in Graham's study and all of
them were handicapped, but they all had accompanying periventricular
leukomalacia (Graham *et al.*, 1987).

The wide spectrum of pathology which can result from a parenchymal
echodensity seen in the first week of life makes it impossible at present to
predict the degree of handicap with any accuracy. This imprecision is the
reason for counselling against the use of ultrasound as a tool for selecting
infants for euthanasia. Future advances, perhaps combining ultrasound
imaging with MRI and spectroscopy and other techniques, may refine our
ability to identify preterm infants who are certain to be severely handicapped in the critical first few days. The likely consequence of this prediction is of such importance that only the highest quality research will suffice
to answer the question.

Conclusion

The dramatic difference in the outcome after GMH–IVH and parenchymal
lesions, whether they are periventricular leukomalacia or porencephalic
cysts, supports the distinction between them, abandoning the concept of a
continuum between four grades of periventricular haemorrhage introduced
by Papile *et al.* (1978). The chance of a normal or an adverse outcome
related to the ultrasound diagnosis in the neonatal period is summarised
in Figs. 12.4 and 12.5. GMH–IVH, unless followed by the rare complication of ventricular enlargement, has an extremely good prognosis and
those with enlarged ventricles may in future be detected early, as may
those patients who have early white matter injury where the dilatation is
mainly due to cerebral atrophy. The current success in reducing the incidence of GMH–IVH is in part due to antenatal steroids and postnatal
surfactant (Rennie, *et al.*, 1996), but this leaves no room for complacency.
Parenchymal brain lesions appear early as echodense areas due to haemorrhage or oedema, and may disappear or evolve into single or multiple cysts.
White matter injury is still an area of active research and further large-scale
studies or even national registries of cases are needed to understand the
natural history of this condition. Such studies would need to document
the incidence, the area affected, the duration of abnormal appearances
requiring repeated ultrasonography for several months after birth, and be
complemented with associated MRI-MRS information and good quality
complete follow-up.

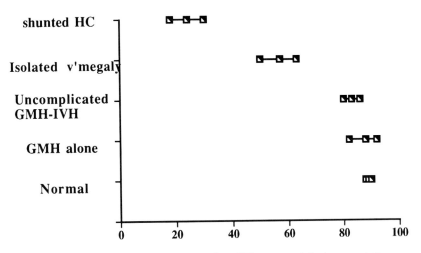

Fig. 12.4. *Chance of normal outcome after different cranial ultrasound diagnoses made in the neonatal period. Shown as percentage with 95% confidence intervals; data from the summary Tables 12.2 to 12.6. HC: hydrocephalus; v'megaly: ventriculomegaly; GMH–IVH: germinal matrix haemorrhage–intraventricular haemorrhage.*

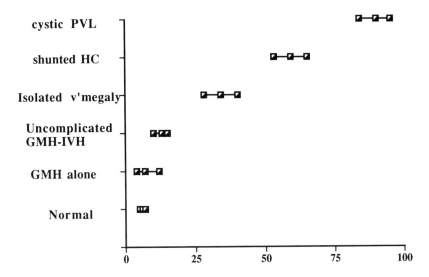

Fig. 12.5. *Chance of major handicap after different cranial ultrasound diagnoses made in the neonatal period. Shown as percentage with 95% confidence intervals; data from the summary Tables 12.2 to 12.6. PVL: periventricular leucomalacia; HC: hydrocephalus; v'megaly: ventriculomegaly; GMH–IVH: germinal matrix haemorrhage–intraventricular haemorrhage.*

References

Achenbach, T.M., Howell, C.T., Aoki, M.F. & Rauh, V.A. (1993) Nine-year outcome of the Vermont Intervention Program for low birth weight. *Pediatrics,* **91**:45–55.

Allan, W.C., Holt, P.J., Sawyer, L.R. Tito, A.M. & Meade, S.K. (1982) Ventricular dilatation after neonatal periventricular haemorrhage–intraventricular haemorrhage. *American Journal of Disease in Childhood,* **136**:589–93.

Allan, W.C., Dransfield, D.A. & Tito, A.M. (1984) Ventricular dilatation following periventricular-intraventricular haemorrhage: outcome at age 1 year. *Pediatrics,* **73**:158–62.

Amiel-Tison, C. & Stewart, A.L. (1989) Follow up studies during the first 5 years of life: a pervasive assessment of neurological function. *Archives of Disease in Childhood,* **64**:496–502.

Appleton, R.E., Lee, R.E.J. & Hey, E.N. (1990) Neurodevelopmental outcome of transient neonatal intracerebral echodensities. *Archives of Disease in Childhood,* **69**:27–9.

Beverley, D.W., Smith, I.S., Beesley, P., Jones, J. & Rhodes, N. (1990) Relationship of cranial ultrasonography, visual and auditory evoked responses with neurodevelopmental outcome. *Developmental Medicine and Child Neurology,* **32**:210–22.

Blackman, J.A., McGuiness, G.A., Bale, J.F. & Smith, W.L. (1991) Large postnatally acquired porencephalic cysts: unexpected developmental outcomes. *Journal of Child Neurology,* **6**:58–64.

Boynton, B.R., Boynton, C.A., Merritt, T.A., Vaucher, Y.E., James, H.E. & Bejar, R.S. (1986) Ventriculoperitoneal shunts in very low birthweight infants with intracranial haemorrhage. Neurodevelopmental outcome. *Neurosurgery,* **18**: 141–5.

Bozynski, M.E.A., Nelson, M.N., Genaze, D., Rosati-Skertich, C., Matalon, T.A.S., Vasan, U. & Naughton, P.M. (1988) Cranial ultrasonography and the prediction of cerebral palsy in infants weighing <1200 grams at birth. *Developmental Medicine and Child Neurology,* **30**:342–8.

Bozynski, M.E.A., DiPietro, M.A., Meisels, S.J., Plunkett, J.W., Burpee, B. & Claflin, C.J. (1990) Cranial sonography and neurological examination of extremely preterm infants. *Developmental Medicine and Child Neurology,* **32**:575–81.

Brothwood, M., Wolke, D., Gamsu, H., Benson, J. & Cooper, D. (1986) Prognosis of the very low birthweight baby in relation to gender. *Archives of Disease in Childhood,* **61**:559–64.

Calame, A., Fawer, C-L., Claeys, V., Arrazola, L., Ducret, S. & Jaunin, L. (1986) Neurodevelopmental outcome and school performance of very low birthweight infants at 8 years of age. *European Journal of Pediatrics,* **145**:461–6.

Catto-Smith, A.G., Yu, V.Y.H., Bakuk, B., Orgill, A.A. & Astbury, J. (1985) Effect of neonatal periventricular haemorrhage on neurodevelopmental outcome. *Archives of Disease in Childhood,* **60**:8–11.

Chalmers, I. & Altman, D.G. (1995) *Systematic Reviews.* London: BMJ Publishing Group.

Cooke, R.W.I. (1987a) Early and late cranial ultrasonographic appearances and outcome in very low birthweight infants. *Archives of Disease in Childhood,* **62**:931–7.

Cooke, R.W.I (1987b) Determinants of major handicap in post haemorrhagic hydrocephalus. *Archives of Disease in Childhood*, 62:504–7.

De Vries, L.S., Dubowitz, L.M.S., Dubowitz, V., Kaiser, A., Lary, S., Silverman, M., Whitelaw, A. & Wigglesworth, J.S. (1985) Predictive value of cranial ultrasound in the newborn baby: a reappraisal. *Lancet*, ii:137–40.

De Vries, L.S., Connell, J.A., Dubowitz, L.M.S, Oozeer, R.C. & Dubowitz, V. (1987) Neurological, electrophysiological and MRI abnormalities in infants with extensive cystic leukomalacia. *Neuropediatrics*, 18:61–6.

De Vries, L.S., Regev, R., Pennock, J.M., Wigglesworth, J.S. & Dubowitz, L.M.S. (1988) Ultrasound evolution and later outcome of infants with periventricular densities. *Early Human Development*, 16:225–33.

De Vries, L.M.S., Eken, P., Groenendaal, F., Van Haastert, I.C. & Meiners, L.C. (1993) Correlation between the degree of periventricular leukomalacia diagnosed using cranial ultrasound and MRI later in infancy in children with cerebral palsy. *Neuropaediatrics*, 24:263–8.

Dykes, R.D., Dunbar, B., Lazzara, A. & Ahmann, P. (1989) Posthaemorrhagic hydrocephalus in high risk preterm infants: natural history, management and long-term outcome. *Journal of Pediatrics*, 114:611–18.

Eken, P., van Niuwenhuizen, O., van der Graaf, Y., Schalij-Delfos, N.E. & de Vries, L.S. (1994) Relation between neonatal cerebral ultrasound abnormalities and cerebral visual impairment. *Developmental Medicine and Child Neurology*, 36:3–15.

Escobar, G.J., Littenberg, B. & Pettiti, D.B. (1991) Outcome among surviving very low birthweight infants: a meta-analysis. *Archives of Disease in Childhood*, 66:204–11.

Etches, P.C., Ward, T.F., Bhui, P.S., Peters, K.L. & Robertson, C.M. (1987) Outcome of shunted posthemorrhagic hydrocephalus in premature infants. *Pediatric Neurology*, 3:136–40.

Farmer, S.F. & Harrison, L.M. (1991) Plasticity of central motor pathways in children with hemiplegic cerebral palsy. *Neurology*, 41:1505–10.

Fawer, C.-L., Diebold, P. & Calame, A. (1987) Periventricular leucomalacia and neurodevelopmental outcome in preterm infants. *Archives of Disease in Childhood*, 62:30–6.

Fawer, C.-L. & Calame, A. (1991) Significance of ultrasound appearances in the neurological development and cognitive abilities of preterm infants at 5 years. *European Journal of Pediatrics*, 150:515–20.

Fazzi, E., Lanzi, G., Gerardo, A., Ometto, A., Orcesi, S. & Rondini, G. (1992) Neurodevelopmental outcome in very low birthweight infants with or without periventricular haemorrhage and/or leucomalacia. *Acta Paediatrica Scandinavica*, 81:808–11.

Fazzi, E., Orcesi, S., Caffi, L. Ometto, A., Rondini, G., Telesca, C. & Lanzi, G. (1994) Neurodevelopmental outcome at 5–7 years in preterm infants with periventricular leukomalacia. *Neuropediatrics*, 25:134–9.

Fernell, E. & Hagberg, G. (1993) Infantile hydrocephalus in preterm VLBWI – a nationwide Swedish cohort 1979–1988. *Acta Paediatrica Scandinavica*, 82:45–8.

Gaffney, G., Squier, M.V., Johnson, A., Flavell, V. & Sellers, S. (1994) Clinical associations of prenatal ischaemic white matter injury. *Archives of Disease in Childhood*, 70:F101–F106.

Gluckman, P.D. (1992) When and why do brain cells die? *Developmental Medicine and Child Neurology*, 34:1010–21.

Goldstein, R.B., Filly, R.A., Hecht, S. & Davis, S. (1989) Noncystic 'increased' periventricular echogenicity and other mild cranial sonographic abnormalities: predictors of outcome in low birth weight infants. *Journal of Clinical Ultrasound*, 17:553–62.

Graham, M., Levene, M.I., Trounce, J.Q. & Rutter, N. (1987) Prediction of cerebral palsy in very low birthweight infants. *Lancet*, ii:593–6.

Graziani, L.J., Pasto, M. & Stanley, C. *et al.*, (1985) Cranial ultrasound and clinical studies in preterm infants. *Journal of Pediatrics*, 106:269–76.

Graziani, L.J., Pasto, M., Stanley, C., Pidcock, F., Desai, H., Desai, S., Branca, P. & Goldberg, B. (1986) Neonatal neurosonographic correlates of cerebral palsy in preterm infants. *Pediatrics*, 78:88–95.

Graziani, L.J., Mitchell, D.G., Kornhauser, M,. Pidcock, F.S., Merton, D.A., Stanley, C. & McKee, L (1992) Neurodevelopment of preterm infants: neonatal neurosonographic and serum bilirubin studies. *Pediatrics*, 89:229–34.

Greisen, G., Petersen, M.B., Pedersen, S.A. & Baekgaard, P. (1986) Status at two years in 121 very low birthweight survivors related to neonatal intraventricular haemorrhage and mode of delivery. *Acta Paediatrica Scandinavica*, 75:24–30.

Grether, J.K., Cummins, S.K. & Nelson,K.B. (1992) The California cerebral palsy project. *Pediatric and Perinatal Epidemiology*, 6:339–51.

Guit, G.L., Van De Bor, M., Den Ouden, L. & Wondergem, J.H.M. (1990) Prediction of neurodevelopmental outcome in the preterm infant: MR staged myelination compared with cranial ultrasound. *Pediatric Radiology*, 175:107–9.

Guzzetta, F., Shackleford, G.D., Volpe, S., Perlman, J.M. & Volpe, J.J. (1986) Periventricular intraparenchymal echodensities in the premature newborn: critical determinant of neurologic outcome. *Pediatrics*, 78:995–1006.

Hagberg, B., Hagberg, G., Olow, I. & Von Wendt, L. (1989) The changing panorama of cerebral palsy in Sweden. V: The birth year period 1979–82. *Acta Paediatrica Scandinavica*, 78:283–90.

Hagberg, B., Hagberg, G. & Olow, I. (1993) The changing panorama of cerebral palsy in Sweden. VI. Prevalence and origin during the birth year period 1983–86. *Acta Paediatrica Scandinavica*, 82:387–93.

Hansen, N.B., Kopechek, J., Miller, R.R., Menke, J.A. & Cordero, L. (1989) Prognostic significance of cystic intracranial lesions in neonates. *Developmental and Behavioral Pediatrics*, 10:129–33.

Hellema, H. (1992) Dutch issue guidelines on handicapped babies. *British Medical Journal*, 305:1312–13.

Hislop, J., Dubowitz, L.M.S., Kaiser, A., Singh, M.P. & Whitelaw, A. (1988) Outcome of infants shunted for posthaemorrhagic ventricular dilatation. *Developmental Medicine and Child Neurology*, 30:451–6.

Hungerford, J., Stewart, A. & Hope, P. (1986) Ocular sequelae of preterm birth and their relation to ultrasound evidence of cerebral damage. *British Journal of Ophthalmology*, 70:463–8.

International Neonatal Network (1993) The CRIB (Clinical Risk Index for Babies) score: a tool for assessing initial neonatal risk and comparing performance of neonatal intensive care units. *Lancet*, 342:193–8.

Janowsky, J.S. (1986) Outcome of perinatal brain damage. *Developmental Medicine and Child Neurology*, 28:375–89.

Jongmans, M., Henderson, S., De Vries, L.S. & Dubowitz, L.M.S. (1993) Duration of periventricular densities in preterm infants and neurological outcome at 6 years of age. *Archives of Disease in Childhood*, 69:9–13.

Kaiser, A. & Whitelaw, A. (1985) Cerebrospinal fluid pressure during posthaemorrhagic ventriculomegaly in newborn infants. *Archives of Disease in Childhood*, **60**:920–4.

Kitchen, W.H., Ford, G.W., Murton, L.J., Rockards, A.L., Ryan, M.M., Lissenden, J.V., de Crespigny, L.C. & Fortune, D.W. (1985) Mortality and two-year outcome of infants of birthweight 500–1500 g: relationship with neonatal cerebral ultrasound data. *Australian Pediatric Journal*, **21**:253–9.

Kitchen, W.H., Ford, G.W., Rickards, A.L., Doyle, L.W., Kelly, E. & Murton, L.J. (1990) Five-year outcome of infants of birthweight 500–1500 grams: relationship with neonatal ultrasound data. *American Journal of Perinatology*, **7**:60–5.

Leichty, E.A., Gilmor, R.L., Bryson, C.Q. & Bull, M.J. (1983) Outcome of high-risk neonates with ventriculomegaly. *Developmental Medicine and Child Neurology*, **25**:162–8.

Levene, M.I. (1981) Measurement of the growth of the lateral ventricles in preterm infants with real time ultrasound. *Archives of Disease in Childhood*, **56**:900–40.

Levene, M.I. (1990) Cerebral ultrasound and neurological impairment: telling the future. *Archives of Disease in Childhood*, **65**:469–71.

Levene, M.I., Dowling, S., Graham, M., Fogelman, K., Galton, M. & Phillips, M. (1992) Impaired motor function (clumsiness) in five-year-old children: correlation with neonatal ultrasound scan. *Archives of Disease in Childhood*, **67**:687–90.

Lucas, A., Morley, R., Cole, T.J. *et al.* (1990) Early diet in preterm babies and developmental status at 18 months. *Lancet*, **335**:1477–81.

Maher, J. E., Cliver, S.P., Goldernberg, R. L., Davis, R.O., Copper, R.L. & the March of Dimes Multicenter Study Group. (1994) The effect of corticosteroid therapy in the very premature infant. *American Journal of Obstetrics and Gynaecology*, **170**: 869–73.

Monset-Couchard, M., de Bethemann, O., Radvanyi-Bouvet, M-F., Papin, C., Bordarier, C. & Relier, J.P. (1988) Neurodevelopmental outcome in cystic periventricular leukomalacia: 30 cases. *Neuropediatrics*, **19**:124–31.

Mutch, L.M.M., Johnson, M.A. & Morley, R. (1989) Follow up studies: design, organisation and analysis. *Archives of Disease in Childhood*, **64**:1394–402.

Ng, P.C. & Dear, P.R.F. (1990) The predictive value of a normal ultrasound scan in the preterm baby – a meta-analysis. *Acta Paediatrica Scandinavica*, **79**:286–91.

Oka, A., Belliveau, M.J., Rosenberg, P.A. & Volpe, J.J. (1993) Vulnerability of oligodendroglia to glutamate: pharmacology, mechanisms and prevention. *Journal of Neuroscience*, **13**:1441–3.

Palmer, P., Dubowitz, L.M.S., Levene, M.I. & Dubowitz, V. (1982) Developmental and neurological progress of preterm infants with intraventricular haemorrhage and ventricular dilatation. *Archives of Disease in Childhood*, **57**:748–53.

Paneth, N., Rudelli, R., Kazam, E. & Monte, W. (1994) Brain damage in the preterm infant. *Clinics in Developmental Medicine* No 131. London: MacKeith Press.

Pape, K.E. & Wigglesworth, J.S. (1979) *Haemorrhage, Ischaemia and Perinatal Brain. Clinics in Developmental Medicine*, Nos. 69/70. London: Spastics International Medical Publications.

Papile, L.-A., Burstein, J., Burstein, R. & Koffler, H. (1978) Incidence and evolution of subependymal and intraventricular hemorrhage: a study of infants with birthweight <1500g. *Journal of Pediatrics*, **92**:529–34.

Patterson, P.H. (1993) Neuronal differentiation factors/cytokines and synaptic plasticity. *Neuron*, **10**:123–37.

Pharoh, P.O.D., Cooke, T., Rosenbloom, L. & Cooke, R.W.I. (1987) Trends in birth prevalence of cerebral palsy. *Archives of Disease in Childhood*, **62**:379–84.

Pharoh, P.O.D., Cooke, T., Cooke, R.W.I. & Rosenbloom, L. (1990) Birthweight specific trends in cerebral palsy. *Archives of Disease in Childhood*, **65**:602–6.

Pharoh, P.O.D., Stevenson, C.J., Cooke, R.W.I. & Stevenson, R.C. (1994) Clinical and subclinical deficits at 8 years in a geographically defined cohort of very low birthweight infants. *Archives of Disease in Childhood*, **70**:264–70.

Pidcock, F.S., Graziani, L.J., Stanley, C., Mitchell, D.G. & Merton, D. (1990) Neurosonographic features of periventricular echodensities associated with cerebral palsy in preterm infants. *Journal of Pediatrics*, **116**:417–22.

Pierrat, V., Eken, P., Duquennoy, C., Rousseau, S. & De Vries, L.S. (1993) Prognostic value of early somatosensory evoked potentials in neonates with cystic leukomalacia. *Developmental Medicine and Child Neurology*, **35**:683–90.

Pike, M.G., Holmstrom, G., de Vries, L.S., Pennock, J.M., Drew, K.J., Sonksen, P.M. & Dubowitz, L.M.S. (1994) Patterns of visual impairment associated with lesions of the preterm infant brain. *Developmental Medicine and Child Neurology*, **36**:849–62.

Pinto-Martin, J.A., Riolo, S., Cnaan, A., Holzman, C., Susser, M. & Paneth, N. (1995) Cranial ultrasound prediction of disabling and nondisabling cerebral palsy at age two in a low birthweight population. *Pediatrics*, **95**:249–54.

Rademaker, K.J., De Vries, L.S. & Barth, P.G. (1993) Subependymal pseudocysts: ultrasound diagnosis and findings at follow up. *Acta Paediatrica Scandinavica*, **82**:394–9.

Rennie, J.M., Wheater, M. & Cole, T.J. (1996) Antenatal steroid administration is associated with an improved chance of intact survival in preterm infants. *European Journal of Paediatrics*, **155**:576–9.

Scher, M.S., Dobson, V., Carpenter, N.A. & Guthrie, R.D. (1989) Visual and neurological outcome of infants with periventricular leukomalacia. *Developmental Medicine and Child Neurology*, **31**:353–65.

Scottish Low Birthweight Study Group (1992a) The Scottish Low Birthweight Study: I Survival, growth, neuromotor and sensory impairment. *Archives of Disease in Childhood*, **67**:675–81.

Scottish Low Birthweight Study Group. (1992b) The Scottish Low Birthweight Study. II. Language attainment, cognitive status and behavioural problems. *Archives of Disease in Childhood*, **67**:682–6.

Shankaran, S., Keopke, T., Woldt, E., Bedard, M.P., Dajani, R., Eisenbrey, A.B. & Canady, A. (1989) Outcome after posthemorrhagic ventriculomegaly in comparison with mild hemorrhage without ventriculomegaly. *Journal of Pediatrics*, **114**:109–14.

Shortland, D., Levene, M.I., Trounce, J.Q., Ng, Y. & Graham, M. (1988) The evolution and outcome of cavitating periventricular leukomalacia in infancy. A study of 46 cases. *Journal of Perinatal Medicine*, **16**:241–7.

Sinha, S.K., D'Souza, S.W., Rivlin, E. & Chiswick, M.L. (1990) Ischaemic brain lesions diagnosed at birth in preterm infants: clinical events and developmental outcome. *Archives of Disease in Childhood*, **65**:1017–20.

Stanley, F.J. & Watson, L. (1992) Trends in perinatal mortality and cerebral palsy in Western Australia, 1967–1985. *British Medical Journal*, **304**:1658–63.

Stephenson, T. & Barbor, P. (1995) Ethical dilemmas of diagnosis and inter-

232

vention. In *Fetal and Neonatal Neurology and Neurosurgery*, ed. M.I. Levene & R.J. Lilford, pp. 709–18. Edinburgh: Churchill Livingstone.

Stewart, A.L. (1992) Follow up studies. In *Textbook of Neonatology*, ed. N.R.C. Roberton, pp. 49–74. Edinburgh: Churchill Livingstone.

Stewart, A.L., Reynolds, E.O.R., Hope, P.L., Hamilton, P.A., Baudin, J., Costello, A.M. de L., Bradford, B.C. & Wyatt, J.S. (1987) Probability of neurodeveopmental disorders estimated from the ultrasound appearance of brains of very preterm infants. *Developmental Medicine and Child Neurology*, 29:3–11.

Szymonowicz, W., Yu, V.Y.H., Bajuk, B. & Astbury, J. (1986) Neurodevelopmental outcome of periventricular haemorrhage and leukomalacia in infants 1250g or less at birth. *Early Human Development*, 14:1–7.

TeKolste, K.A., Bennett, F.C. & Mack, L.A. (1985) Follow up of infants receiving cranial ultrasound for intracranial haemorrhage. *American Journal of Disease in Children*, 139:299–303.

Tudehope, D.I., Masel, J., Mohay, H., O'Callaghan, M., Burns, Y., Rogers, Y. & Williams, G. (1989) Neonatal cranial ultrasonography as predictor of 2 year outcome of very low birthweight infants. *Australian Pediatric Journal*, 25:66–71.

Van de Bor, M., Veerlove-Vanhorick, S.P., Baerts, W., Brand, R. & Ruys, J.H. (1988) Outcome of periventricular-intraventricular haemorrhage 2 years of age in 484 very preterm infants admitted to 6 neonatal intensive care units in the Netherlands. *Neuropaediatrics*, 19:183–5.

Van de Bor, M., Guit, G.L., Schreuder, A.M., Wondergem, J. & Vielvoye, G.J. (1989a) Early detection of delayed myelination in preterm infants. *Pediatrics*, 84:407–11.

Van de Bor, M., Van Zeben-van der Aa, T.M., Veerlove-Vanhorick, S.P., Brand, R. & Ruys, J.H. (1989b) Hyperbilirubinaemia in preterm infants and neurodevelopmental outcome at 2 years of age: results of a national collaborative study. *Pediatrics*, 83:915–20.

Van de Bor, M., den Ouden, L. & Guit, G.L. (1992) Value of cranial ultrasound and magnetic resonance imaging in predicting neurodevelopmental outcome in preterm infants. *Pediatrics*, 90:196–9.

Van de Bor, M., Ens-Dokkum, M., Schreuder, A.M., Veen, S., Brand, R. & Veerlove-Vanhorick, S.P (1993) Outcome of periventricular-intraventricular haemorrhage at five years of age. *Developmental Medicine and Child Neurology*, 35:33–41.

Ventriculomegaly Trial Group (1990) Randomised trial of early tapping in neonatal posthaemorrhagic ventricular dilatation. *Archives of Disease in Childhood*, 65:3–10.

Ventriculomegaly Trial Group (1994) Randomised trial of early tapping in neonatal posthaemorrhagic ventricular dilatation: results at 30 months. *Archives of Disease in Childhood*, 70:F129–F136.

Weindling, A.M., Rochefort, M.J., Calvert, S.A., Fok, T.-F. & Wilkinson, A. (1985) Development of cerebral palsy after ultrasonographic detection of periventricular cysts in the newborn. *Developmental Medicine and Child Neurology*, 27:800–6.

Weisglas-Kuperus, N., Baerts, W., Fetter, W.P.F. & Sauer, P.J.J. (1992) Neonatal cerebral ultrasound, neonatal neurology and perinatal conditions as predictors of neurodevelopmental outcome in very low birthweight infants. *Early Human Development*, 31:131–48.

Weisglas-Kuperus, N., Heersema, D.J., Baerts, W., Fetter, W.P.F., Smorkovsky, M., van Hof-van Duin, J. & Sauer, P.J.J. (1993) Visual functions in relation with neonatal cerebral ultrasound, neurology and cognitive development in very low birthweight children. *Neuropaediatrics*, **24**:149–54.

Wheater, M. & Rennie, J.M. (1994) Poor prognosis after prolonged ventilation for bronchopulmonary dysplasia. *Archives of Disease in Childhood*, **71**:F210–F211.

Whitaker, A., Johnson, J., Sebris, S., Pinto, J., Wasserman, G., Kairam, R., Shaffer, D. & Paneth, N. (1990) Neonatal cranial ultrasound abnormalities: association with developmental delay at age one in low birthweight infants. *Developmental and Behavioural Pediatrics*, **11**:253–60.

Wigglesworth, J.S. (1989) Plasticity of the developing brain. In *Perinatal Brain Lesions*, ed. K.E. Pape & J.S. Wigglesworth, pp. 253–69. Cambridge, Mass: Blackwell Scientific Publications.

Williams, M.L., Lewandowski, L.J., Coplan, J. & D'Eugenio, D.B. (1987) Neuro-developmental outcome of preschool children born preterm with and without intracranial haemorrhage. *Developmental Medicine and Child Neurology*, **29**:243–9.

Index

Page numbers in italics indicate figures.

A-mode 4, *5*
abscess, brain 171
accuracy, of measurements 33–4
acetazolamide 95
acoustic impedance 2
acoustic shadow 2, 35
Acuson 21, 22, 27
Advanced Technology Laboratories
    (ATL) 21, 22
Aicardi's syndrome 179
alarms 31
aliasing 11, 12–13
    in colour Doppler 14
allopurinol 137
Aloka 21, 22
American Institute of Ultrasound in
    Medicine (AIUM) 14, 32
aminophylline 95–6
analgesia 96
aneurysms
    congenital 110, 189–93
    vein of Galen 189–93
angled parasagittal section *40*, 48–51
antepartum haemorrhage *148–9*, 150,
    200
anterior cerebral artery 71, *72*, Plate
    5.1
    coronal view 39, *41*
    reversed flow 86
apnoea 29, 31
arachnoid cysts 185, *188*, *190–1*
archiving, picture 26–7
Arnold-Chiari malformation 51, 182,
    183–4
artefacts 34–7
arterio-venous malformations 110
asphyxia, birth 89–90, 150, 196
atrophy, cerebral, *see* cerebral atrophy
attenuation 2, 7
audio signals 71
audio tape recorders 76

autoregulation, cerebral blood flow
    (CBF) 83–6
axial resolution 7
axial section 51

B & K Medical 22
B-mode 4–6
babies
    handling 28–31
    hygiene 31
    monitoring equipment 29–31
    positioning 28–9
basal ganglia *42*, 43
basilar artery 43, 48, *72*
BBS Medical Electronic 22
birth asphyxia 89–90, 150, 196
blood
    transfusion 83
    viscosity 83
blood pressure 83–6, 126
blush, peritrigonal 45–8
boundary *3*, 9
bradycardia 29, 31
brain death 90
brainstem 43, *44*
'bright brain' 197
British Medical Ultrasound Society 32

caffeine 95–6
calcarine fissure 58
calcification 170, *171*
    thalamic 170, 171–5, 193
    vascular 193
carbon dioxide 82–3
carotid arteries *72*
catheters, intraventricular 165, 166–7
caudate nucleus
    coronal views *42*, 43, *44*
    parasagittal views 48, *50*
cavitation 15–16
cavum septum pellucidum 51, *53*

cavum septum pellucidum (*cont.*)
  bleeding into 115
  coronal views 40, *42, 44*
cavum vergae 40, 48, 51
  bleeding into 115
cephalhaematoma 110
cerebellum
  agenesis/hypoplasia 182
  coronal views 43–5, *46*
  haemorrhage 116
  sagittal views 48, *49*
cerebral arteries 71, *72*
cerebral atrophy
  causes 157
  prognosis 212, 220
  vs hydrocephalus 155–9
cerebral blood flow (CBF)
  absent 90
  autoregulation 83–6
  reverberating pattern, in brain death 90
  reversed diastolic *75*, 86–7, 89
  validation studies 81, 82
cerebral blood flow velocity (CBFV)
  calculations 76
  drug studies 91–6
  in hypoxic ischaemic encephalopathy 196
  in newborn brain injury 89–91
  normal values 77–9, 80–1
  in patent ductus arteriosus 86–7
  physiological changes affecting 82–7
  sources of error 80
  validation studies 81–2, 84–5
  variability 87–8
cerebral oedema 197, *198–9*
cerebral palsy
  epidemiology 210, *211*, 212
  lesions predicting 212–13, 224–5, 226
  in periventricular leukomalacia 142, 144, 213, 224–5
  thalamic lesions and 197
cerebral peduncles 51
cerebrospinal fluid
  aspiration (ventricular tap) 165, 219
  raised pressure, *see* intracranial pressure, raised
choroid plexus 48–51
  cysts 45, 185, *191*
  glomus of 45, *47*, 48
  haemorrhage 118–19
  papilloma 189

chromosomes, ultrasonic disruption 16
cingulate sulcus 56, *57*
  midline sagittal view 48, *49*
  in preterm infants 56, *57*–61, 62
cisterna magna 43, 48, *49*, 51
  enlarged 161
citrobacter meningitis 171
coagulopathies 107–8, 126
'cobblestone' appearance 62
colour Doppler 14, Plate 1.1
  congenital vascular lesions 189
  safety guidelines 17
colour flow mapping (CFM) 14
compact disc 26–7
congenital infections 170, *171–2*
congenital malformations 177–93
continuous wave (CW) Doppler 10, 73
contrast resolution 8
'convexity cerebral haemorrhage' 113, *115*
coronal sections 38, 39–48
  anterior horns of lateral ventricles 40–3
  brain scoring *61*
  frontal lobes 39–40, *41*
  quadrigeminal cisterns 43–5, *46*
  third ventricle 43, *44*
  trigone 45–8
corpus callosum
  agenesis 179–82
  coronal views 40, *42*
  lipomas 189
  parasagittal views 48, *49*
coupling agent, *see* jelly, ultrasound
cystic disorders, congenital 183–9
cysts
  arachnoid 185, *188, 190–1*
  choroid plexus 45, 185, *191*
  Dandy–Walker 185, *186–7*
  leptomeningeal 111, *114*, 185
  parenchymal 212, 224
  in periventricular leukomalacia *142*, 143–51
  porencephalic, *see* porencephalic cysts
  subependymal 128, *130*
cytomegalovirus, congenital 170, *171–2*, 193

Dandy–Walker cysts 185, *186–7*
Dandy–Walker malformation 182, 185
Dandy–Walker variant 185
database, ultrasound equipment 20–1

death
  brain 90
  of co-twin *in utero* 110, 136
demodulation 10
Diagnostic Sonar 23
Diasonics Sonotron (Vingmed) 22
diazepam 96
digital audio tape recorders 76
disability 213
dopamine 86
Doppler effect 1, 9–10
Doppler equation 10
Doppler ultrasound 1–2, 9–14, 71–96
  analysis of information 74–80
  clinical studies 82–8
  colour, *see* colour Doppler
  drug studies 91–6
  duplex, *see* duplex Doppler systems
  in hydrocephalus/ventriculomegaly
    89, 91, 92–4, 165
  in hypoxic ischaemic encephalopathy
    196
  mean velocity calculations 76
  in newborn brain injury 89–91
  normal values 77–9, 80–1
  safety guidelines 17
  signal optimisation 71–4
  signal processing 13–14
  signal recording 27–8, 76
  validation studies 81–2, 84–5
  waveform indices 76–80
drugs, Doppler studies 91–6
ductus arteriosus, patent 73–4, *75*, 86–
  7, 136
duplex Doppler systems 11, *12*, 71–3
  maximum velocity limit 11
duty cycle 32
Dynamic Imaging 21, 22

electroencephalography (EEG) 196
encephalomalacia, multicystic *146–8*,
  149–51, 200–1, *202–7*
encephalopathy
  clinical presentation 196
  hypoxic ischaemic, *see* hypoxic
    ischaemic encephalopathy
endotracheal tube fixation systems 28–
  9, *30*
energy 2, 31–2
  maximum acceptable levels 14–15, 32
  see also power, acoustic
equipment, ultrasound 20–37
  artefacts 34–7
  guidelines 21–5

image storage 25–8
major manufacturers 22–5
on-line database 20–1
quality control 33–4
safe use 28–33
Escherichia coli meningitis 116, *174*,
  175
euthanasia, passive 214
examination, cranial ultrasound 38–9
exposure time 32, *33*
extracorporeal membrane oxygenation
  (ECMO) 116

falx cerebri, bleeding into 115
'figure of three' effect 48, *49*
fissures, maturational changes 56–70
'flares', periventricular 48, 137–42, 223
fontanelle, anterior 38
footprint 6
foramen of Munro 43, *44*
Fourier transform 13–14, 74
fourth ventricle 43, *46*
Fraunhofer field 8
frequency 2
Fresnel field 8
frontal lobes
  coronal view 39–40, *41*
  height measurement 56
frontal sulcus 58

Gammex RMI 23, 34
GE Medical Systems 23
gel, *see* jelly, ultrasound
germinal matrix (subependymal)
    haemorrhage 123, 127
  accuracy of diagnosis 127
  incidence *124*, *125*
  prognosis 219, 220, *227*
  ultrasound appearance 128–9, *130*
germinal matrix haemorrhage-
    intraventricular haemorrhage
    (GMH-IVH) 123–34, 155, 215
  accuracy of diagnosis 126–7
  aetiology and prevention 126
  classification 127, 128
  incidence and timing 124–6
  prognosis 219, 221, 226, *227*
  ultrasound appearances 128–34
gestational age
  brain score and *62*
  cerebral blood flow velocity and 81
  normal brain appearances and 56–70
  periventricular leukomalacia and *125*
  see also preterm infants

GLANCE 20–1
gliosis 138
globus pallidus *42*, 43
glutamate 214
growing skull fracture 111, *114*, 185
gyri
    maturational changes 56–70
    secondary 61, 62

haemorrhage
    antepartum *148–9*, 150, 200
    cerebellar 116
    choroid plexus 118–19
    'convexity cerebral' 113, *115*
    extracerebral 110–15
    fetal, postnatal effects 107–10
    germinal matrix, *see* germinal matrix
        haemorrhage
    germinal matrix-intraventricular, *see*
        germinal matrix haemorrhage-
        intraventricular haemorrhage
    intracerebral 115–19
    intraventricular, *see* intraventricular
        haemorrhage
    parenchymal, *see* parenchymal
        haemorrhage/lesions
    periventricular, *see* periventricular
        haemorrhage
    in preterm infants 123–34
        accuracy of diagnosis 126–7
        aetiology and prevention 126
        classification 127, 128
        history/terminology 123–4
        incidence and timing 124–6
    subarachnoid 110, 113, *115*
    subdural 110–11, *112–13*
    subependymal, *see* germinal matrix
        haemorrhage
    subgaleal 110
    thalamic 115–16, *117*
haemorrhagic arterial cerebral
    infarction 110, 116, *118*
haemorrhagic disease of newborn 159
hand washing 31
handicap
    definition 213
    lesions predicting 212–13
    in preterm survivors, *see* preterm
        infants, handicap in
hats 28–9, *30*
hearing impairment 211
heating effects 15
hemiplegia 133–4, 210
Hewlett Packard 21, 23

holoprosencephaly 177, *178–80*
human platelet antigen 1 (HPA1) 107
hydranencephaly 157–9, 183–5
hydrocephalus 155
    arachnoid cysts and 185, *188*, *190–1*
    in Arnold-Chiari malformation 182,
        183
    causes 157
    congenital 108, 157–9
    Doppler studies *89*, 91, 92–4, 165
    external 155, *156*, *204*
    normal pressure 155
    posthaemorrhagic 157, *158*
    postnatal 157
    prenatally acquired 157
    prognosis 220–24, 224, *227*
    progressive 156, 165, 219–23
    vs cerebral atrophy 155–9
    see also ventriculomegaly
hydrops fetalis 108
hygiene 31
hyperbilirubinaemia 136
hypotension 110, 136, *147*, 150
hypoxic ischaemic encephalopathy
    196–207
    cerebral oedema in 197, *198–9*
    middle cerebral artery infarction 197
    thalamic lesions 197, *200*
    white matter injury 200–1, *202–7*

image
    archiving 26–7
    display methods 4–6
    storage/recording 25–8, 39, 76
immature infants, *see* preterm infants
impairment 213
impedance, acoustic 2
incubators, imaging babies in 28–9, *30*
indomethacin 95
infarction
    cerebral arterial 110, 116, *118*, 197
    cerebral venous 123
infections 170–5
    congenital 170, *171–2*
    neonatal 171–5
inferior temporal sulcus *57*, 61
insula 51, 56, 58
intensity, power 32
    exposure time and 32, *33*
    spatial average (I_{sa}) 32
    spatial peak (I_{sp}) 32
    spatial peak temporal average (I_{spta})
        32
internal capsule 39, *41*, *44*

interpeduncular cistern 43, 48, *49*
intracerebral haemorrhage 115–19
intracranial pressure, raised
    Doppler studies 89–90
    prognosis 219
    signs 156
    ventriculomegaly in 155, 165
intraparenchymal haemorrhage, *see*
        parenchymal haemorrhage/
        lesions
intravenous lines 29
intraventricular catheters 165, 166–7
intraventricular haemorrhage 116, 123
    accuracy of diagnosis 127
    classification 127, 128
    incidence *124*, *125*
    parenchymal haemorrhage with, *see*
        parenchymal haemorrhage/lesions
    ultrasound appearance 129–30, *131*,
        132
    see also germinal matrix
        haemorrhage-intraventricular
        haemorrhage (GMH-IVH)
ischaemic lesions, in preterm infants
    134–51
island of Reil 56

jelly, ultrasound 28, 31
    lack of 34–5
Joubert's syndrome 182

KeyMed 22, 23
Kodak 23
Kontron 23
Kretztechnik 23

lateral resolution 7–8
lateral sulcus 56
lateral ventricles
    coronal views 40–3, 45–8
    normal variations 51
    parasagittal views 48, *50*
learning difficulties 213
leptomeningeal cyst 111, *114*, 185
leukomalacia, periventricular, *see*
        periventricular leukomalacia
Levene ventricular index 155, 159,
        161, *162*, *163*
line density 7
linear array 4–6
    phased 6
lipoma, corpus callosum 189
lissencephaly 182–3
lumbar puncture 165

malformations, congenital 177–93
massa intermedia 48
mature infants, *see* term infants
measurements, accuracy of 33–4
mechanical sector 6
meningitis 116, 171–5
micro-streaming 15
midazolam 96
middle cerebral artery (MCA) 71, *72*,
        Plate 5.2
    coronal view 40–3
    infarction *118*, 197
midline sagittal section *40*, 48, *49*
    brain scoring 60
Miller–Dieker syndrome 183
mirror image production 35, *36*
monitoring
    preterm/ill infants 29–31
    ventriculomegaly 165–7
morphine 96
multicystic encephalomalacia
    (encephalopathy) *146–8*, 149–51,
        200–1, *202–7*
myelomeningocoele (spina bifida) 182,
        184

necrotising enterocolitis 136
neonatal units 28–31
neural tube disorders 182
neurological handicap, *see* handicap
neuronal proliferation disorders 182–3
noise, 7
    excessive 35–7
nurses, neonatal 28
Nyquist limit 11

occipital cortex 48
occipital gyri 58
oedema, cerebral 197, *198–9*
orbital ridge 39, *41*
owl's eye 157
oxygen
    saturation monitors 29–31
    tension 83
    therapy 29

Panasonic 24
pancuronium 96
papilloma, choroid plexus 189
parasagittal sections 38–9, *40*, 48–51
    angled 48–51
    brain scoring *59–60*
    tangential 51, *52*, 59
    see also midline sagittal section

parenchymal haemorrhage/lesions 123–4, *135*
  classification 127, 128
  hypoxic ischaemic 200–1, *202–7*
  incidence *124*, *125*
  prognosis 213, 224–7
  ultrasound appearances 131–4, *135*
  see also germinal matrix haemorrhage; periventricular leukomalacia
parents 28
parietal sulcus 58
parieto–occipital sulcus 56, *57*
  midline sagittal view 48, *49*
  in preterm infants 58, 61
patent ductus arteriosus 73–4, *75*, 86–7, 136
pericallosal artery 71, *72*
peritrigonal blush 45–8
periventricular 'flares' 48, 137–42, 223
periventricular haemorrhage 123–34
  prognosis 220, 221
  ultrasound appearances 128–34
  see also germinal matrix haemorrhage-intraventricular haemorrhage
periventricular halo 45–8
periventricular leukomalacia 134–51
  aetiology and prevention 136–7
  diagnosis and classification 137
  gestational age and *125*
  grade I and II 137–42
  grade III (with multiple cysts) *142*, 143–9
  grade IV (subcortical cysts/ multicystic encephalopathy) *146–8*, 149–51, 200–1, *202–7*
  haemorrhagic 123, 131–2
  history and terminology 134
  incidence and timing *124*, *125*, 134–6
  prognosis 142, 144, 213, 214, 223–5, *227*
  ultrasound diagnosis 137–51
  ventriculomegaly in 155
phantoms 34
phased linear array 6
phenobarbitone 96, 126
Philips 24
PI, *see* Pourcelot index
Pie Medical 21, 24, *26*
piezoelectric crystals 4
pons 48, *49*
porencephalic cysts 133–4, *135*

in utero haemorrhage causing 107, *109*
  prognosis 225–6
positioning of babies 28–9
post-Rolandic fissure 58
posterior communicating artery *72*
Pourcelot index (of resistance) (PI) 76–80
  carbon dioxide tension and 82
  in hydrocephalus *89*, 91, 92–4
  in newborn brain injury *89*, 90, 91
  normal values 77–9, 80
power, acoustic 31–3
  definition 32
  Doppler systems 73
  exposure time and 32, *33*
  measuring output 32–3
  see also energy
pressure, acoustic 32, 33
preterm infants
  cavum septum pellucidum 51, *53*
  CBF autoregulation 86
  Doppler studies
    brain-injured infants 90
    normal infants 77–9, 80–1
  haemorrhagic lesions 123–34
  handicap in
    after normal scans 215–18
    epidemiology 210–12
    future prospects 214–15
    lesions predicting 212–14
    in specific lesions 219–26
  handling 28–31
  ischaemic lesions 134–51
  monitoring equipment 29–31
  normal brain appearances 56–70
    23–24 weeks 56, *63*
    25–26 weeks 57–8, *64*
    27–28 weeks 58, *65*
    29–31 weeks 58–61, *66*
    32–33 weeks 61–2, *67*
    35–36 weeks 62, *68*
  passive euthanasia 214
  prognosis 210, 215–26
  subarachnoid spaces 51–4
  vascular lesions 123–51
printers 25–6
probes, *see* transducers
prognosis 210, 215–26
prosencephalic disorders 177–82
Proteus meningitis 171
pseudocysts, subependymal 189, *192*, 219
pulmonary blood flow 91
pulsatility index 80

pulse-echo 4
pulse repetition frequency (PRF) 11,
    13
pulsed wave (PW) Doppler 10, 32
putamen *42*, 43, *44*

quadrigeminal cisterns
    coronal views 43–5, *46*
    sagittal views 48, *49*
quadriplegia 210
quality control 33–4

range-gated 11
real-time imaging 4–6
reflection 1, *3*
refraction 1, 2, *3*
resolution 6–8
    axial 7
    contrast 8
    lateral 7–8
    temporal 8
respiration, cerebral blood flow velocity
    (CBFV) and 87–8
respiratory distress syndrome 126
reverberation echoes 34–5
ring echos 34–5
rubella, congenital 170

safety
    in handling babies, parents, neonatal
        nurses 28–31
    of ultrasound 14–17, 31–3
        epidemiological surveys 16
        physical effects 15–16
        reports/recommendations on 16–
            17, 32
    in use of ultrasound 28–33
sagittal section, midline, *see* midline
    sagittal section
sample volume 11
scattering 2
schizencephaly 182
scoring systems, brain 56, *59–61*
sedation 96
seizures 86
septo-optic dysplasia 177, 178
septum pellucidum
    agenesis of 177–9
    failure of fusion 178–9
shadow, acoustic 2, 35
shock waves 15, 32
Siel Imaging Equipment Ltd 21, 24
Siemens 24
skull fracture, growing 111, *114*, 185

sleep state 80–1
slit ventricle syndrome 167
sonar 1
sonogram 74, *75*
Sony 24
spastic diplegia 134, 210, 212
speckle, excessive 35–7
spectral analysis 11, 13–14, 74, *75*
spina bifida (myelomeningocoele) 182,
    184
steroids, antenatal 124, 215
streaming 15–16
stroke, *see* infarction
subarachnoid haemorrhage 110
    focal (haematoma) 113, *115*
    generalised 113
subarachnoid spaces 51–4
subcortical cystic leukomalacia *146–8*,
    149–51
subdural effusions *174*, 175
subdural haemorrhage 110–11, *112–13*
subependymal cyst 128, *130*
subependymal haemorrhage, *see*
    germinal matrix haemorrhage
subependymal pseudocysts 189, *192*,
    219
subgaleal haemorrhage 110
sulci
    maturational changes 56–70
    tertiary 62
sunsetting 156
superior temporal sulcus *57*, 58
suppression 8–9
surfactant 91–5
Swift Technologies 25, 27
Sylvian fissure
    coronal views 43, *44*
    maturational changes 56, *57*
    parasagittal view 51, *52*
    in preterm infants 56, 57, 58, 62

tangential parasagittal section 51, *52*
    brain scoring *59*
tela choroidea 48, *49*
temporal bone
    axial section at 51
    Doppler ultrasound via 71, *73*
temporal resolution 8
temporal sulci *57*, 58, 61
term infants
    normal appearances 62–70
    normal flow velocity values 77–9,
        80–1
    vascular lesions 107–19

test objects 34
thalamus
  calcification 170, 171–5, 193
  coronal view 45, *46*
  haemorrhage 115–16, *117*
  hypoxic ischaemic lesions 197, *200*
  parasagittal view 48, *50*
thiopentone 96
third ventricle
  coronal view 43, *44*
  sagittal views 48, *49*
thrombocytopaenia, alloimmune 107,
  108
time, exposure 32, *33*
time-gain compensation (TGC) 8–9
Toshiba 21, 25
toxoplasmosis, congenital 170
transducers (probes) 4–6
  Doppler 10–11
  hygiene 31
  resolution 7
transfusion, blood 83
'trapped' ventricle syndrome 167, 171
tumours, congenital 189
turbulent flow 14
twin pregnancy 110, 136

ultrasound
  basic principles 2, *3*
  discovery 1–2
  display methods 4–6
  Doppler, *see* Doppler ultrasound
  echo location 4
  equipment, *see* equipment,
    ultrasound
  improving the image 8–9
  limits of resolution 6–8
  physical and biological effects 14–17
Ultrasound Equipment Evaluation
  Project (UEEP) database 20–1, 25

vascular calcification 193
vascular lesions
  congenital 189–93
  immature infants 123–51
  mature infants 107–19
  see also haemorrhage
vein of Galen
  aneurysms 189–93
  blood flow velocities 81
velocity

cerebral blood flow, *see* cerebral
  blood flow velocity
  mean, calculation 76
  of moving target, estimating 9–14
  of ultrasound transmission 2
venous blood flow velocities 81
ventilation, artificial 87–8, 136
ventricle:brain width ratio 159
ventricles, cerebral *45*
  area measurements 161–4
  enlarged, *see* ventriculomegaly
  linear measurements 159–61
  measurement 159–65
  normal variations 51
  'trapped' 167, 171
  volume measurements 164–5
ventricular catheters 165, 166–7
ventricular index of Levene 155, 159,
  161, 162, 163
ventricular tap 165, 219
ventriculitis 171, *173*
ventriculo-peritoneal shunts 165, 219–
  24
ventriculomegaly 155–67
  causes 155–9
  Doppler studies *89*, 91, 92–4, 165
  in intraventricular haemorrhage 127,
    128, 130
  in meningitis 171
  monitoring 165–7
  in periventricular leukomalacia 155
  prenatal haemorrhage causing 107,
    108–10
  prognosis 219–24, *227*
  progressive *vs* non-progressive 165
  ultrasound assessment 159–65
  see also hydrocephalus
video recorders 27–8, 39
views, standard 38–54
Vingmed 22
viscosity, blood 83
visual handicap 211, 213
vitamin K 126, 159

wall-thump filter 13, 73
wavelength 2
white matter injury
  hypoxic ischaemic 200–1, *202–7*
  prognosis 223–8
  see also parenchymal haemorrhage/
    lesions
World Health Organisation (WHO)
  212, 213